ENDORSEMENTS

"Given the success of this performance and its impact on our community of patients, survivors and providers, SMIL hopes to continue our support of the mission of 'A 2nd Act' through future collaborations."

John Freeman, Director of Sales & Marketing
Scottsdale Medical Imaging

"What an inspiration these women are to others struggling with cancer, being able to take a tragedy/hardship in life and see the blessings from it. Remarkable women making a difference in this world!"

Kelly B. Huey MSW, LCSW, OSW-C
Director of Integrative Services & Social Work
Ironwood Cancer & Research Centers

"The grace, humor and strength with which these women face their personal battles with cancer should serve to inspire and enlighten anyone facing a similar battle."

Jim Brewer
Executive Director
Arizona Chapter, The Leukemia & Lymphoma Society

a 2nd Act

CANCER SURVIVORS CHANGING THE QUESTION FROM "**WHY ME?**" TO "**WHAT NEXT?**"

A2ndAct.org

A 2nd Act:
Cancer Survivors Changing the Question from "Why Me?" to "What Next?"

Volume 1: Edition 3

Printed in the United States of America.

Requests for information
and permission should be addressed to
A 2nd Act Publishing
www.A2ndAct.org
info@A2ndAct.org

Cover design and book layout by
La Verne Abe Harris
Cover Photography by Alex Hamrick
of LarryJohnWright.com

ISBN-13: 978-1543151749

To order additional copies,
or to buy books in quantity, please visit
www.A2ndAct.org

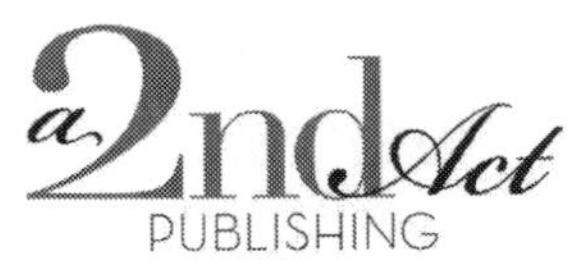

DEDICATION

If you're going through hell, keep going.
-Winston Churchill

As anyone who's ever had cancer, or watched someone battle cancer, can attest to, the disease is exactly the kind of hell dear Winston had in mind. The key is to keep going. That's true whether it refers to treatment or life in general. And neither of those are solo journeys.

This book, then, is dedicated to the women whose stories lie within; the brave women who created 2nd Acts. It's also dedicated to the millions of cancer survivors and their loved ones who might be touched by their words.

Lastly, this book is dedicated to all of the sponsors, donors, and grantors who, through their generosity, have allowed us to bring these survivors' stories to stage and share them with others.

TABLE OF CONTENTS

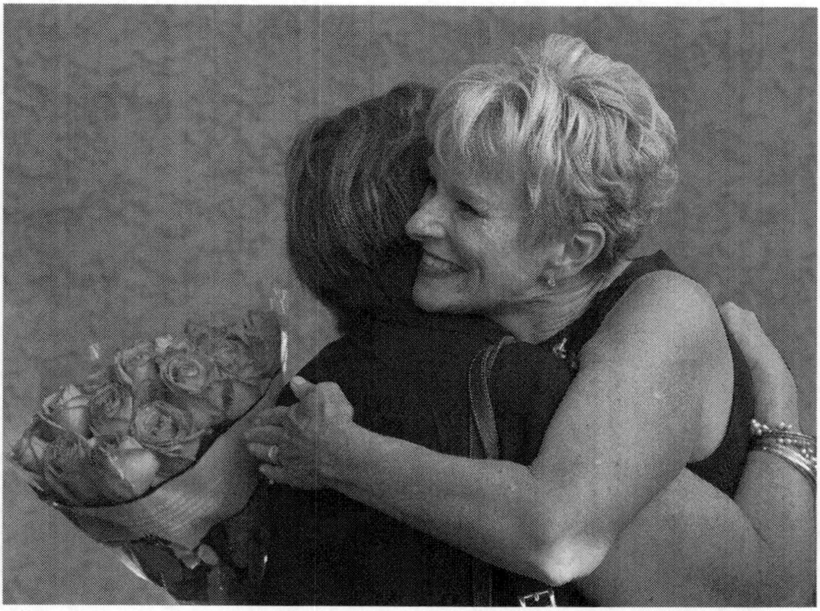

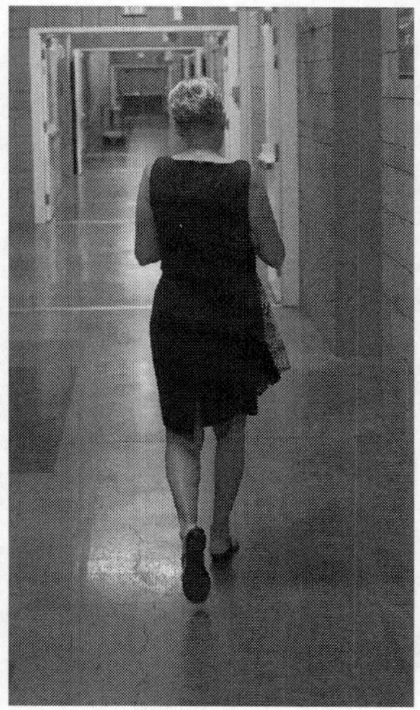

Judy is off to the next show...

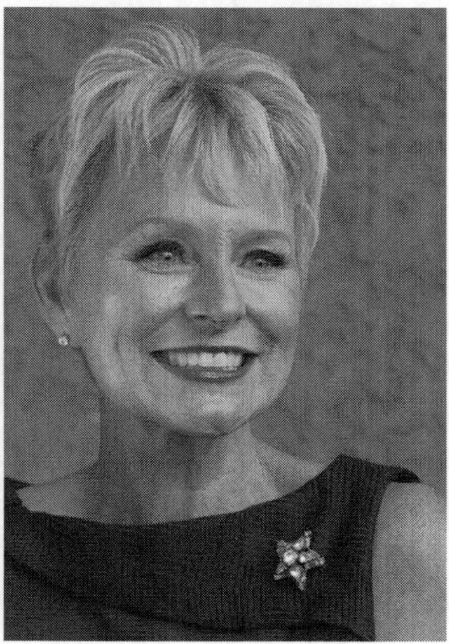

Judy Pearson, Founder

INTRODUCTION

Any woman cancer survivor can tell you precisely where she was the moment she heard the words that changed her life forever: "You have cancer." A tsunami of doctors and drugs, procedures and scans, hurry up and wait ensue. Then, after months, maybe years, the waters of frenetic activity part. The big day arrives. Treatment is over.

But wait! There was safety and structure in that treatment. As survivors, we are suddenly struck by the realization there is no Humpty Dumpty moment when all the pieces of our lives will be put back together, rebuilding the person we once were. Rather, we often find ourselves still dragging the carcass of our ill-ness behind us. Whether we're told we have no evidence of disease, or that we must live with our cancer, what will fill the holes now that the diagnosis and treatment stages have leveled off? How do we push "play" on a once-paused life? What was it all for?

I know this first hand, as do the more than eight million women survivors of all cancers in America. The cancer journey will forever be a part of our story. It is a story in two acts. Act 1 was our life before cancer. Now our 2nd Act must begin.

I'm a writer by profession, and my non-fiction work makes me a researcher as well. I stumbled on statistics supporting the idea that "healing is helping" while working on a book in my pre-cancer days. When I came across that same volunteering research as my post-cancer self, I realized that this most important element of healing – giving to others in some way, any way – was missing from the checklist of other support organizations.

Furthermore, whether aware of that research or not, women survivors across the country are taking their lives back by doing amazing things in their 2nd Acts. They're using their newly realized gifts of life and experience to give back to the greater good. They're making sense of their cancer journey and finding its purpose in their lives. I've had the honor of meeting hundreds of them face to face. And that's when my brain's lightbulb switched to the "on" position - and A2ndAct.org was born!

A2ndAct.org supports and celebrates these women survivors by giving them a platform from which to share their stories: "A 2nd Act: Survivorship Takes the Stage." These curated stage performances feature eight to 10 women survivors, local to their performance city, using the centuries old craft of storytelling. They are ordinary women inspiring their audiences to create their own 2nd Acts, regardless of what life challenge might lie before them.

The money raised from these performances (and the purchase of this book, and other fundraisers) allows us to make micro-grants to women survivors, ready to reenter their lives and begin their 2nd Acts. Most importantly, the money stays in the cities where it was raised.

Within the pages of this book, you'll find the amazing stories of the women who have graced our stage, along with our hope that you, too, will be inspired to overcome whatever obstacle might be blocking your path. We further hope that you'll share what you learn with others who might also need to create a 2nd Act.

As performances occur, we'll add those cast members' stories in new editions of this book. The beauty of the printed word is that, whether one lives in a performance city or not, the opportunity for inspiration is just fingertips away.

I thank you for your support, as woman by woman, city by city, we change survivors' life focus from "Why me?" to "What next?"

Judy Pearson
Cancer Survivor and Founder
A2ndAct.org

AMERICAN WOMEN AND CANCER

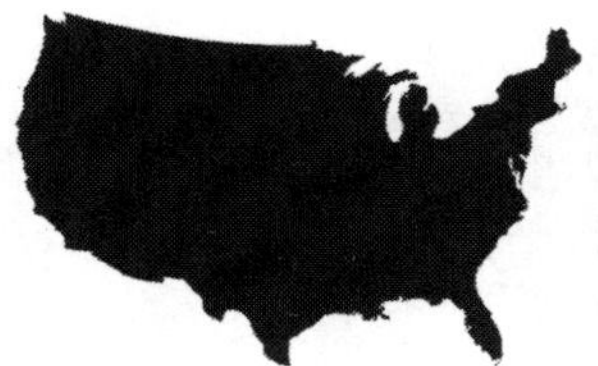

An estimated **843,820** women in the United States will be diagnosed with some form of cancer in 2016. There are nearly **8 MILLION** women survivors in the US.

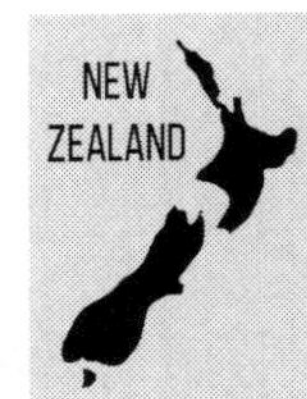

That's a number greater than the population of New Zealand, Hong Kong, or Norway.

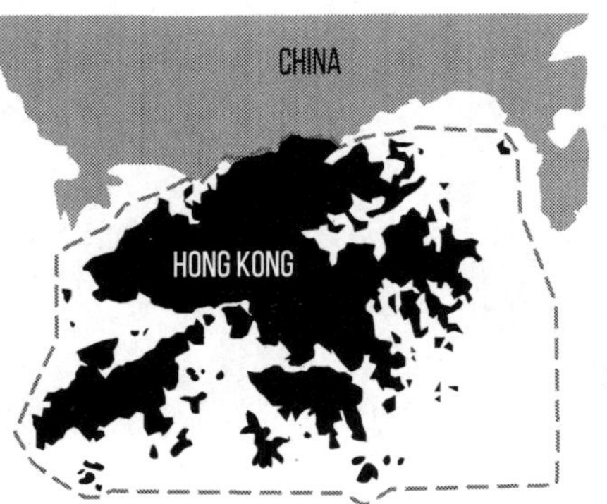

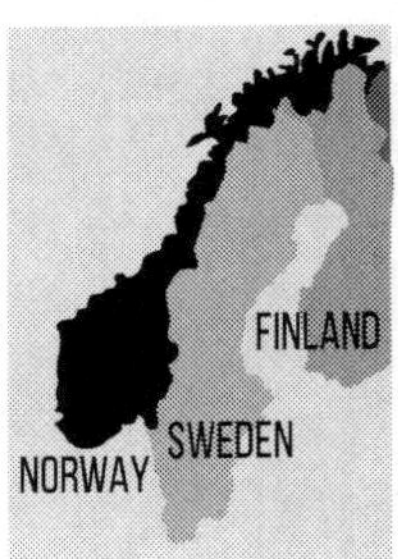

It's also greater than the **combined** populations of Luxembourg (bordered by Belgium, Germany and France), Jamaica and Puerto Rico.

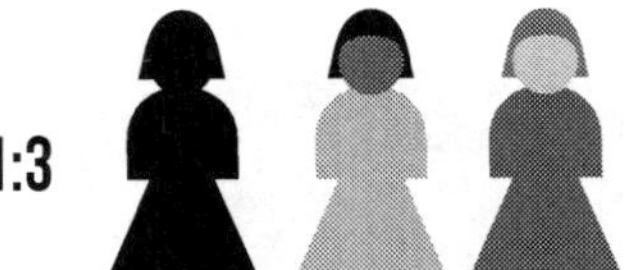

One in three women will be diagnosed with some form of cancer during their lifetime. If not you, you will know her. She may be your friend, neighbor, mother, sister or even your daughter.

La Verne Abe Harris

Sources: American Cancer Society Statistics 2016, Wikipedia

Cancer doesn't end when treatment does.
Even if the disease is cured tomorrow,
women survivors would still face challenges
they never expected:

CANCER'S COLLATERAL DAMAGE

Financial Toxicity, Careers, Relationships, and Fear

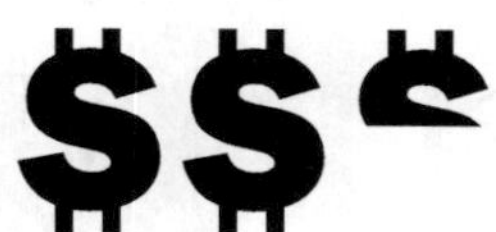

FINANCIAL TOXICITY

Cancer survivors file for bankruptcy **2.5 TIMES** more often than the rest of the population. Fred Hutchinson Cancer Research Center coined the phrase "financial toxicity" of cancer.

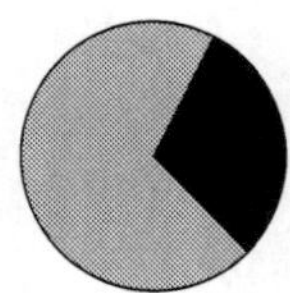

CAREERS

30% of women cancer survivors in a University of Michigan study say they have had difficulty returning to their careers.

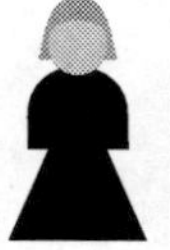

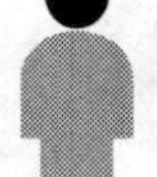
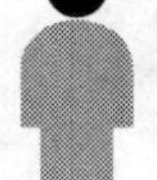

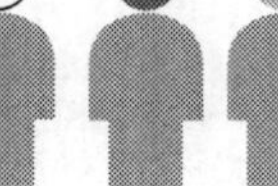

RELATIONSHIPS

Men are **7 TIMES** more likely than women to end a relationship due to significant illness.

FEAR

70% of women survivors fear a recurrence of their cancer.

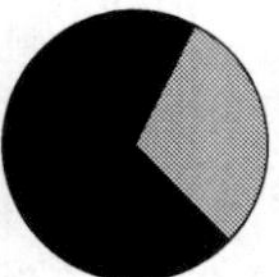

La Verne Abe Harris

Sources: Fred Hutchinson Cancer Research Center, University of Michigan, Huntsman Cancer Institute

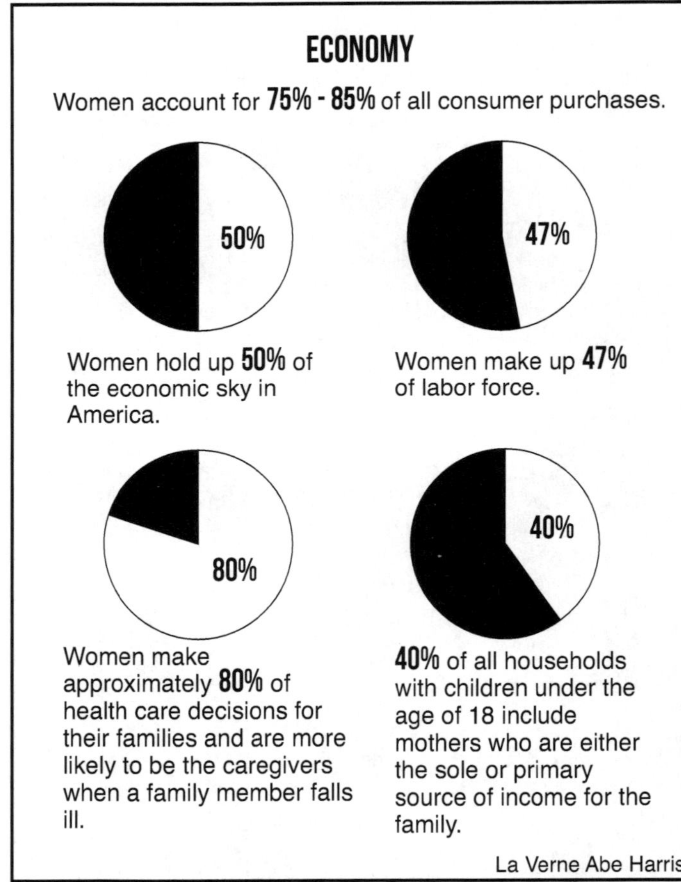

Sources: Pew Research Center Data, 2013; U.S. Department of Labor, 2013; Boston Consulting Group, Nielson, and others

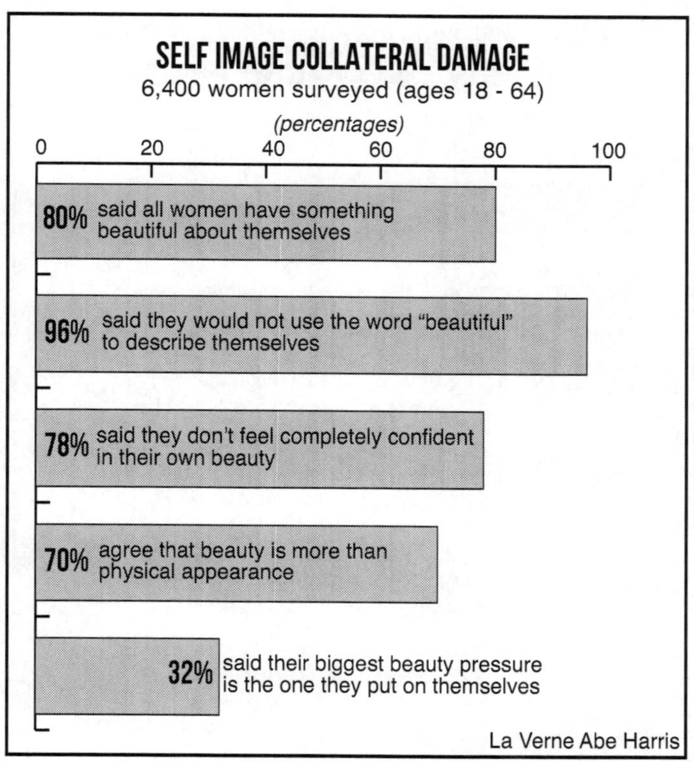

Source: 2015 Dove's Choose Beautiful campaign

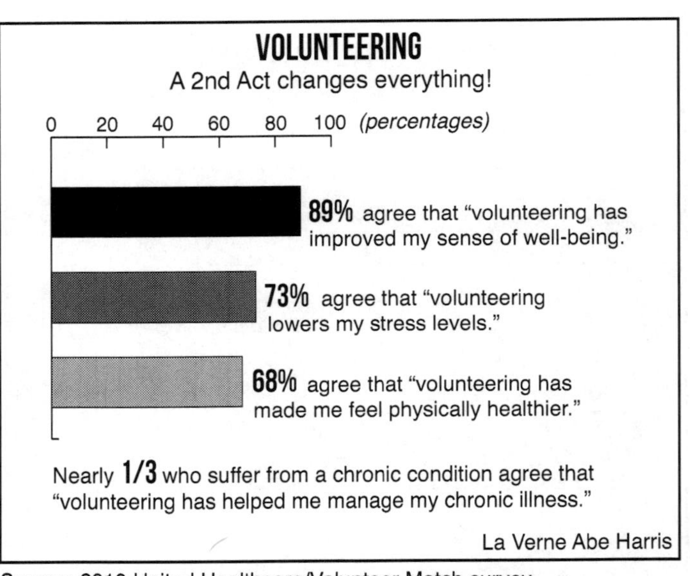

Source: 2010 United Healthcare/Volunteer Match survey of more than 4,500 Americans about volunteering.

THE MISSION AND WORK OF A2NDACT.ORG

Our Mission: Recognizing that helping is healing, we support and celebrate women survivors of ALL cancers using their gifts of time and experience to give back to the greater good.
Our Work: We are survivors helping survivors take their lives back after cancer.

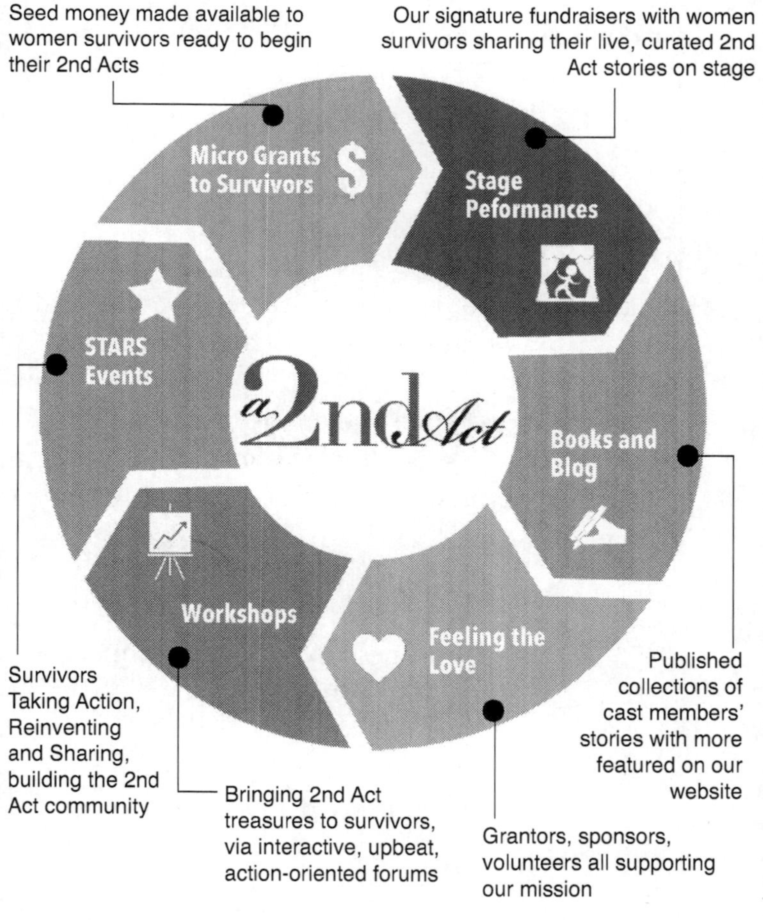

Sources: A 2nd Act

PHOENIX

Like the relentless Arizona summer sun, cancer parches hearts and minds. But cancer didn't stop these women. They shared the stories of their 2nd Acts in the inaugural Valley of the Sun performance.

Sunday, May 22, 2016, 2:00 p.m.
Mesa Arts Center, Mesa, AZ

And as refreshing as rain in the desert, those stories uplifted an audience of nearly 300. Bravo!

This performance was made possible by the generosity of Scottsdale Medical Imaging, Ltd., Ironwood Cancer Research Center, After Breast Cancer Diagnosis, and Caroline Farkas/Berkshire Hathaway Home Services.

Phoenix Photography by Alex Hamrick
of LarryJohnWright.org

Love to Dave Pratt, Emcee
Founder of Star Worldwide Networks

CHAPTER 1

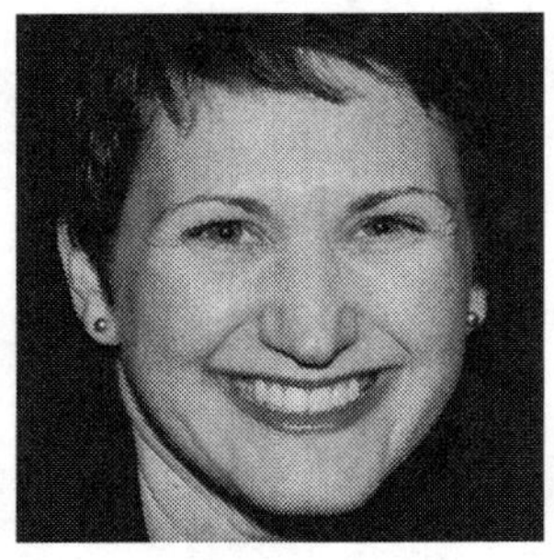

TRACY DIZIERE

Breast Cancer Survivor

A success coach, Tracy Diziere specializes in helping women to discover success strategies so they can make better decisions with newfound clarity and confidence. In guiding women to embrace their authentic strengths and achieve a sense of wholeness, they are able to raise the bar on their own successes.

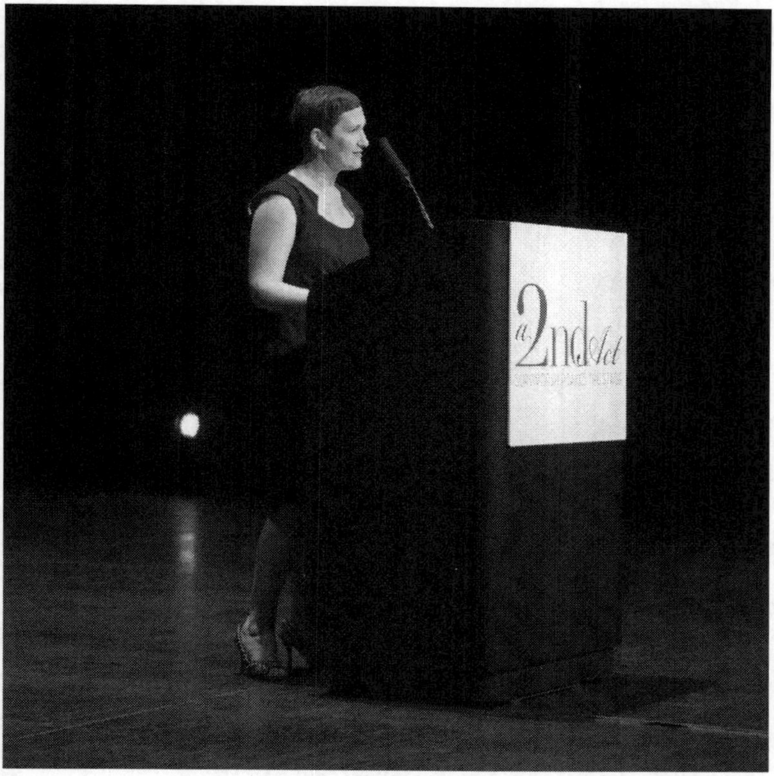

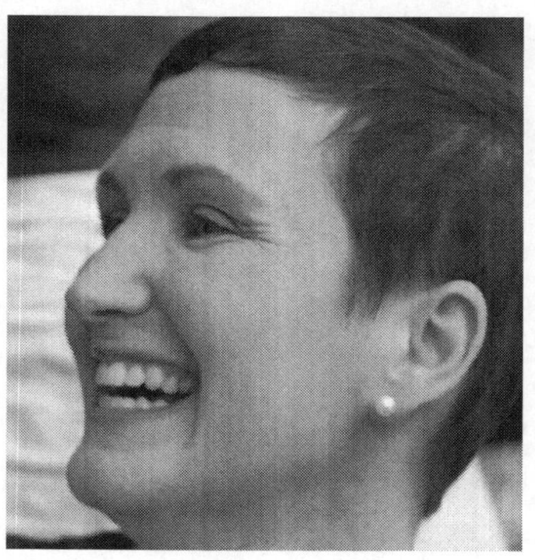

CHAPTER 1: TRACY DIZIERE

On February 13, 2012, I was diagnosed with breast cancer. In conversations, when I tell people this, and I'm sure some of you can probably relate, their reaction is usually one of sorrow or sadness. Their faces drop a little before they can even speak that familiar refrain: "I'm sorry."

But my usual response is "I'm not." In fact, I couldn't be happier about the perspective this experience has given me – and that I'm still here! How about you? Are you happy to be here?

Every woman in this cast is a "cancer success story," but being here is only the first step. I say success story because the term "survivor," for me, creates a divide between those of us here today and others who supposedly just didn't fight hard enough.

Does anyone here think that our mothers, daughters, granddaughters, aunts, nieces, and friends with cancer who have passed on just didn't fight hard enough to survive? So I think it's a mistake to stand here today and disrespect them.

Although I realize this is the popular terminology, I'm hoping we can rise above it . . . and because we already have one accomplishment behind us, I want to help all the success stories out there to focus on what other triumphs we can bring to our lives.

But first, I'd like to talk about how I got here. If you've been through chemo, you know that it's the strangest feeling that the "cure" made you sicker than you felt when you were so-called "sick." And I went through A LOT of strange feelings in the year following my diagnosis. Am I alone here? But it was one of the best years of my life because of the lessons I learned and who I have become.

To explain the impact of this fully, it would help for you to know who I was before cancer or "BC" as I like to say. I wasn't a very positive person. I was suspicious of people, in general. I spent too much time and energy worrying about what other people thought. I placed unnecessary and sometimes unrealistic expectations on myself, and I did not really give myself full permission to be ME at any given moment – especially in workplace or business situations.

I remember feeling like I was expected to constantly adapt to environments with values that did not fit with mine. To complicate matters, I clung too tightly to my own values, which means my hands weren't open for other people.

Despite having read "Don't Sweat the Small Stuff" and all kinds of conflict-management resources, I still "sweated the small stuff!" And I couldn't quite shake the feeling that the enemy was everywhere. Naturally, that caused a lot of stress.

But after cancer, my relationship with people in general – and most importantly with myself – was transformed. I realized how important it is to let others help you. It's important to embrace how connected we all REALLY are when you get down to it.

The life lesson was: We need other people – being comfortable with that is being authentic to the human experience. So is being curious about others' positions and ultra-sensitive to what they might be going through. The truth is we are all vulnerable, so for me that begs the question, why be other than what we are?

This leads to an essential understanding of who I am, how I do business, and how I make decisions. Authenticity – it's at the center of everything I do today. It is the cornerstone of my 2nd Act.

But that doesn't mean I'm the perfect picture of authenticity or the guru on the mountaintop. Authenticity is a journey, not a destination. No one has "arrived." Like yoga, it is a practice, it is a process.

Business and life provide a multitude of tests to learn how to be more authentic, to realize how to do "IT" better, whether the IT is knowing ourselves, loving ourselves and our unique talents, or finding the right language to express ourselves. It takes constant attention. But to find that commonality, within us, within others . . . it is a worthy and rewarding endeavor.

The drive to create the space for people to be authentic – and to give myself permission to be – is what changed for me. It's what propelled me to create my solutions around authentic networking and strengths coaching.

And while helping professionals achieve deeper relationships and be vulnerable or guiding those who might be in "limbo" toward embracing a bigger version of themselves may not seem like a grandiose contribution to society, it is what I am uniquely qualified to do.

We can often solve our own problems because we all have wells of strengths and knowledge to draw from. Bringing authenticity to professional interactions and helping people embrace their strengths to lead more authentic lives are just my small ways of changing the world with the realizations I have had as a result of my cancer journey.

Rebuilding our lives as cancer success stories, we might decide that working for ourselves is our path. We might decide that starting a non-profit is the way to go.

Or we might decide, because we are in a limbo space, that we just need to follow our passions and whisper small yeses to the world for awhile.

My experience with cancer has given me the insight to all this and the strength to pursue my path to happiness, which includes letting it all go, starting with the self-judgment. Instead, I'm choosing to be real and present in my life and my business. That's my challenge to myself, moment by moment, and it's my challenge to you too.

If I could wave a magic wand, I would relieve you of the judgment, self-doubt and pesky insecurities that stand in the way of embracing your authentic selves. And on the other extreme, my wand would allow you to let go of pride and self-importance in exchange for humility and curiosity.

But because I don't have Tinkerbell powers, all I can do is share with you that knowing and honing your strengths and building on your success to date is the greatest gift you can give yourself and others, whether your success comes from a cancer experience or any other life challenge.

You may not think you are cut out to change the world. Or you may think the changes you are making are too small to matter. I'm here to tell you that change is easy and available to you. What is small to you can be life-altering to someone else.

Don't second-guess your value. Take an active step in knowing and embracing your strengths. Make change and celebrate that success. And always remember to keep those hands and hearts open.

CHAPTER 2

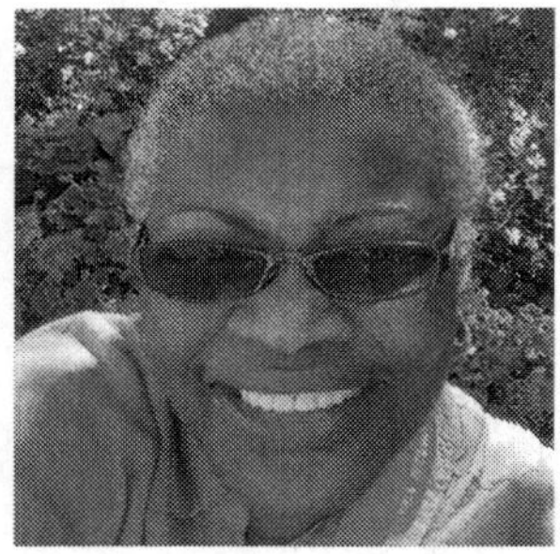

BRENDA JENKINS

Multiple Myeloma Survivor

Brenda Jenkins is an author, inspirational speaker, and consultant. Her topics are leadership, parenting, communication, and living with cancer. Brenda is building an organization – Transparent Teams creating Clarity, Connection, and Community. She believes in the ground root efforts of helping the family starting with Parent Leadership.

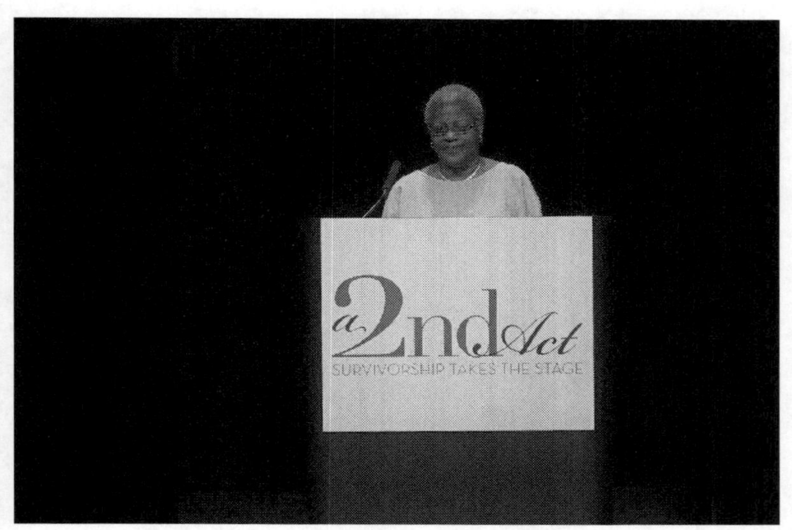

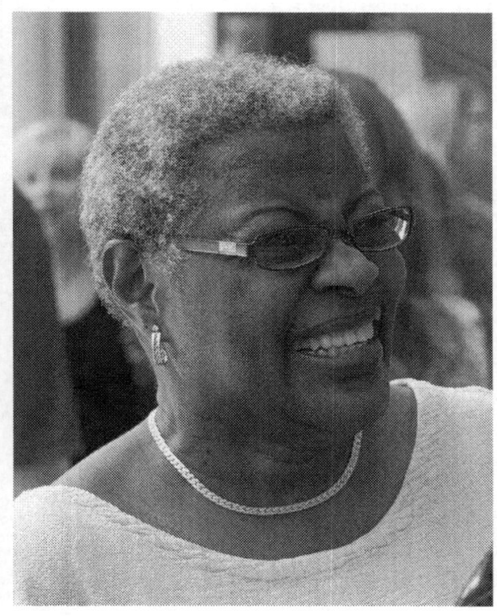

CHAPTER 2: BRENDA JENKINS

I am the mother of four adult children and grandmother to sixteen. And I am a cancer survivor! March 9, 2016, marked my seventh year on this journey with a rare incurable cancer, called multiple myeloma, a cancer of the blood plasma cells.

I've had many treatments, including chemotherapy, radiation, steroids, a few clinical trials, and two stem cell bone marrow transplants. And I have experienced many challenges: weight gain, weight loss, no hair, shingles, neuropathy, bone pain, pneumonia, upper respiratory infection, food poisoning and lots of fatigue.

With God I have overcome it all. This disease is something I will live with the rest of my life. But I choose not to wait on death. Instead, I live every day!

I have weaknesses like everyone else: fatigue, anxiety and the uncertain relapses of this disease. But using my strengths – a love of learning, sharing, speaking, and communicating – I serve others. And I love doing it. It is my 2nd Act.

After my first stem cell bone marrow transplant, I became an advocate for Multiple Myeloma. I speak around the county sharing my journey with other cancer patients, caregivers, and health care professionals.

Then I wondered, do I dare work toward a future endeavor? The answer was clear – Yes! Yes! Yes indeed! So I went back to school in 2010, working on a Doctorate of Education, majoring in Organization Leadership. I expect to finish by the end of this year.

I want to help in the prevention field of child abuse by working with the developers of parent education programs.

As a parent advocate, I'll perform evaluations and assist with the implementation of parent education programs in organizations, including faith based.

Next, in 2013, while I was still living in Michigan, I ran a 10 week campaign raising funds for the Leukemia and Lymphoma Society. They help support blood cancer patients and research, including for Multiple Myeloma. It was a team effort, and our activities included designing an encouraging letter for business support and another for personal support.

We sent those letters to our Christmas card lists, doctors, local businesses and blood cancer pharmaceutical companies. Anyone we had ever had a relationship with, they got a letter! We had so much fun!

The campaign was also part of a contest for the Michigan Leukemia and Lymphoma Society's Woman of the Year. Each dollar raised was a vote. And I won!

I served as patient panel member at the Leukemia and Lymphoma Society cancer educational program. I recruited participants at a health fair to join the "Be a Match" registry for Bone marrow transplants, and spoke at the national survivor's day event in Michigan, as well as at my local church as Cancer Patient advocate.

I have facilitated a parenting workshop at singles events called "Single But Not Alone Parenting." And my story has been featured in the Chicago Defender, and Conquer Magazine.

As part of my legacy, I have also shared my story with StoryCorps, where it is archived at the American Folklife Center at the Library of Congress, Smithsonian Institution's National Museum of African American History and Culture. It's also archived at Virginia Piper Cancer Center in Scottsdale.

Serving and sharing has helped me in my daily walk. Praise God! After six years, I received my second stem cell bone marrow transplant. Praise the Lord I am still here!

I continue speaking and sharing, using social media to share what I have learned about this multiple myeloma, as well as advocating for parents.

I am living happily within my limits, in spite of my challenges. And I have far more blessings than challenges.

I am blessed with new grandchildren, a move here to Arizona, and meeting wonderful people. I have amazing caregivers, family and friends that help and support me. Most importantly I still have the ability to continue learning, speaking and sharing.

My faith is my inner strength. My prayer is that you are enlightened and empowered from my story to live with the challenges in your life. WORK OUT OF YOUR STRENGTHS as you serve others.

CHAPTER 3

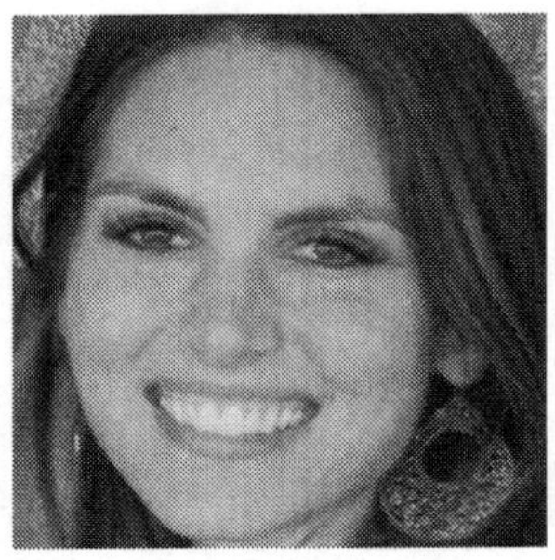

BEKAH PARKER

Hodgkins Lymphoma Survivor

Bekah Parker is from Mesa and the second of five children. She absolutely adores her family! She is a Speech Language Therapist at both an elementary charter school and a private Autism school. She enjoys working out, playing the piano, reading, spending time with friends and family, and traveling

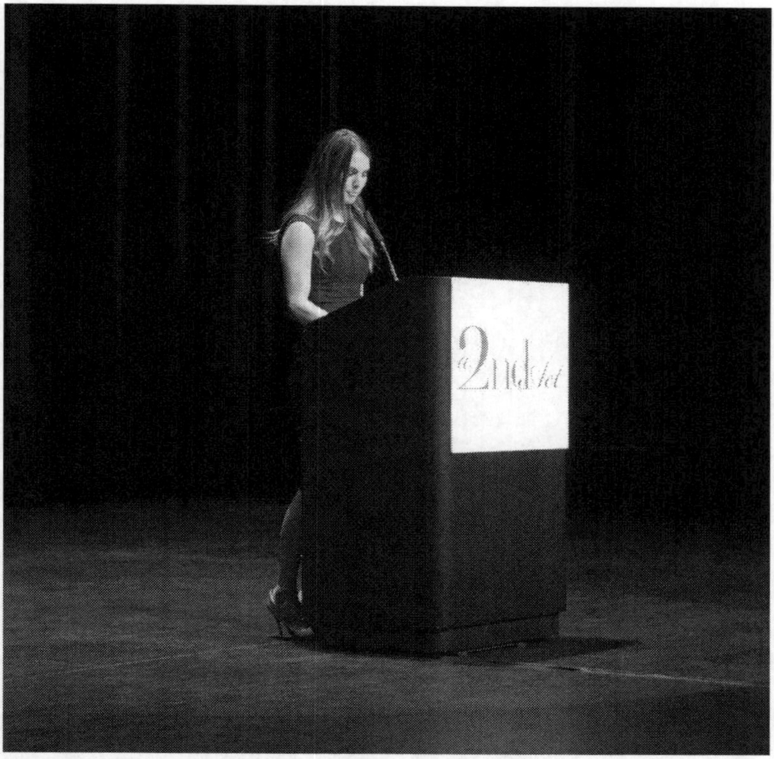

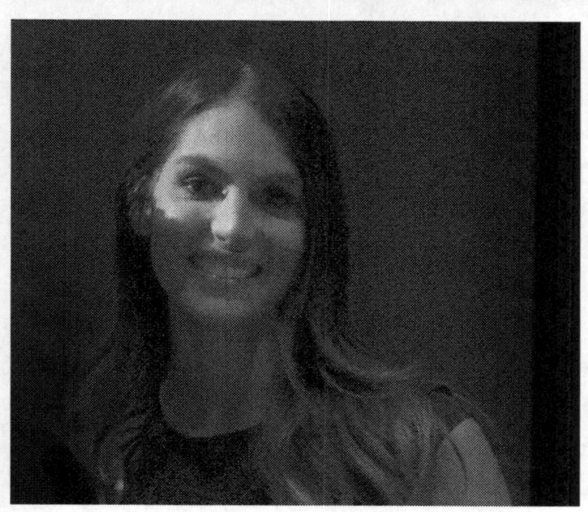

CHAPTER 3: BEKAH PARKER

When I was 18 years old, my life changed forever. After high school I had plans for college and serving a mission for my church. I had lots of friends and I loved spending time with my family. I was just your typical 18-year-old girl.

About four months after I graduated, I started to get really sick. I was tired all the time. It took all I had to get through a day without taking a nap. I was working, going to school, teaching swim lessons, and lifeguarding, so I attributed it to heat exhaustion and a busy schedule.

But it became overwhelming and I told my mom it was time to go to the doctor.

They ran different tests and decided I had Aplastic Anemia. Iron supplements and shots of Procrit didn't seem to help ... at all. After five months, I was getting worse and still had no answers.

By the time Spring Break came, I had dropped out of school, quit my job and was sleeping constantly. A walnut size lump had grown on the side of my throat. I was as white as a ghost and running high fevers along with night sweats and constant itching.

Then came a series of events that I believe were divinely appointed, and I was finally admitted to the hospital with double vision. They never found the cause of the pressure in my brain which was causing the double vision. It went away a day after I was admitted.

I was given two blood transfusions, and the series of testing began, including a bone marrow biopsy, spinal tap, MRI's, CT scans, a biopsy of the lump in my neck and eventually a PET scan. Finally after three days in the hospital and constant testing, we had a diagnosis.

On March 17, 2004, I was diagnosed with Stage 4B Hodgkins Lymphoma. You can never quite explain how your life changes in that moment. I was told that had two more weeks passed without treatment, I would not have survived. I was told I would lose all of my hair, that the chemotherapy would be difficult. I was told that I was very lucky that we had found it just in time.

The chemotherapy started the next day and it continued for nine months. I lost my hair, learned to give myself shots, and was taking up to six to eight medications a day. The doctor's office became a second home. I knew I was in for the fight of my life.

It was long and difficult and painful. But I knew deep down in my heart, that it was all going to be ok. On November 17, I was told the cancer was gone. I no longer needed chemotherapy. I left the doctor's office feeling as if the weight of the world had been lifted from my shoulders.

Since my diagnosis, I will be honest that at first I was paranoid. A headache, meant cancer. A backache meant cancer. An unanticipated sleepless night meant it was back.

I would hold my breathe and my heart would pound each time the doctor would call to tell me the results of follow up testing. But each year I get stronger and stronger. And now, 11 and a half years later, I am still in remission!

Life after cancer has had its own set of challenges. Even though very different, I feel stronger and more confident in my ability to do hard things.

But I feel my 2nd Act has given me the very best life. I graduated from BYU with a degree in Speech Language Pathology. I currently work as a Speech Therapist at Santan Elementary School and Lexington Life Academy, a private autism program.

I have the privilege of working with students with a variety of disabilities. I have always had a heart for the underdog. I have always been super sensitive to kids that feel different or isolated. I believe my sickness only magnified that.

In some part, I can understand how my students feel. I know what it's like to appear different than your peers. I remember watching other 19 year old girls date, go to parties, attend college while I sat in a doctor's office hooked up to machine pouring chemotherapy into my body.

I know what it feels like to not look like those around you. I know what it feels like to get stares and questions on why your life isn't like everyone else's.

My students are special, important, creative, smart, talented, and kind. At my autism school, I work with students who are nonverbal, having sensory processing delays, pragmatic delays, cognitive and academic delays, fine and gross motor delays, unique and special diets, low muscle tone, crippled hands and legs.

But the more I am with them, the more I see them as very special little people who have more to teach ME then I have to teach them. In some ways, they are too special and good to be "typical." I love my students and it is my privilege and opportunity to be a part of their world and to teach them how to be part of ours.

It is a privilege to learn how to combine those two worlds, since in reality they aren't that much different. People tell me that I am making a difference and that I am changing their lives. Perhaps.

But more significantly, they are changing me. In a way it is how I give back. But they are giving me so much more.

My 2nd Act has also involved cancer advocacy. I have been a captain at Relay for Life, where we raised $10,000. Then I created my own non profit called "Bekah's Run for Life." We raise money for blood cancers.

Every day I am blessed to be healthy enough to work out, teach spin classes, and do some personal training.

I am blessed with friends and family. They were a very

steady and sure place for me to fall during my battle. I absolutely love and adore them.

Cancer changes you. But you get to decide HOW it changes you. It changes the way you see life. It changes the way you see yourself.

I used to think that being beautiful meant a lot. But when you are staring in the mirror with no hair, a pale, puffy face and bags under yours eyes, your definition of "beautiful" changes.

Beautiful people are the ones who know pain and sorrow and disappointment. They know what it is like to wake up not knowing if they can survive one more day. They know defeat and intense disappointment. Beautiful people don't just happen.

Cancer doesn't define who I am. I am a survivor of cancer, but aren't we all survivors of some kind? We now get to choose how we will live during our "2nd Acts."

Hopefully we decide to be more kind and loving. A little more soft and accepting of others. A little more compassionate and empathetic towards those we may deem "different."

I hope we decide that our 2nd Act will be more meaningful and worthwhile by giving more of ourselves than asking more of others. May this be our goal and opportunity!

CHAPTER 4

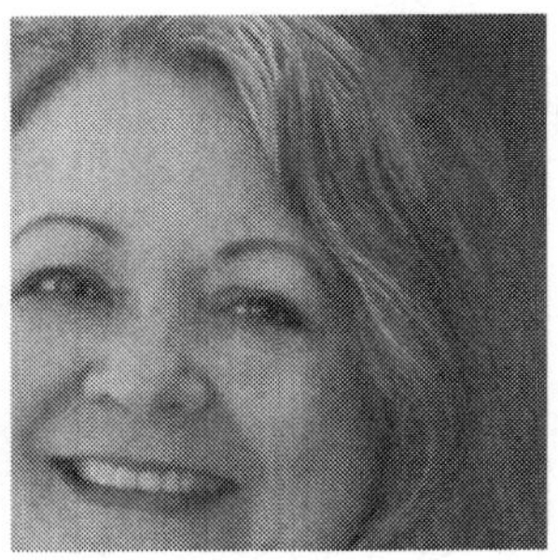

LA VERNE ABE HARRIS

Leukemia Survivor

La Verne Abe Harris is a university professor and artist, who uses her voice, her writing, her humor and her art to inspire, bring joy and heal other cancer patients and those who love them. She lives with love and gratitude for her husband Carl, her children, her grandchildren, and her friends.

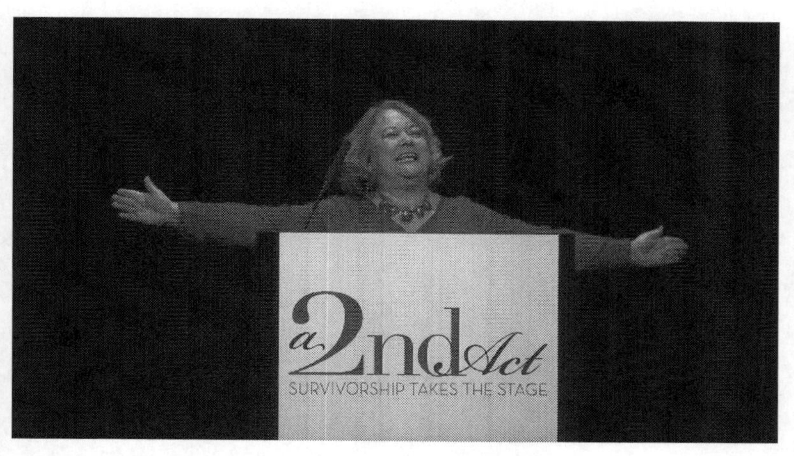
a 2nd Act
SURVIVORSHIP TAKES THE STAGE

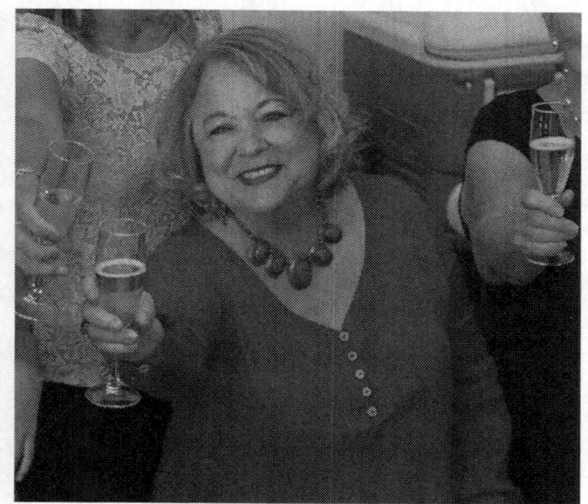

HEY, Big-C! I think from now on I will call you Mr. Buzzkill. I would call you other more irreverent names, but I am, after all, a lady.

I know you remember me. I'm the fat and sassy one – Dr. La Verne, otherwise known as MaMa La Verne. I can't say that I was happy to meet you. But right now we need to talk.

Before YOU disrupted my world, I left Arizona State University and became a tenured professor at Purdue University. I was at the height of my academic career with a research lab and millions of dollars of grant money and YOU stole those dreams from me.

Diagnosis: Leukemia, but further testing to be done. The docs said that maybe I had the "good cancer." Good cancer my ass.

High-risk, they said. Chemo-resistant. So sorry. They said there was nothing they could do. Bone marrow transplant was my only option.

Even better news, I had less than a one percent chance of finding a bone marrow donor, because I happen to be half Japanese and half German. Yep, I'm a rice-schnitzel.

But listen up, Mr. Buzzkill, you didn't discourage this family. When my son had his first daughter, he named her "Hope" for me, because once you have hope, anything is possible.

However, let me add this: "Hope WITHOUT ACTION is for sissies!" So I did my research. I became a proactive patient and I applied to be a participant in a clinical trial with an experimental drug that is now FDA approved. I became the lab rat.

The funny thing is that I have spent my entire life avoiding drugs, that is, until YOU came along. Ironically, I now go for my drug run to the East Coast every three months. Mr. Buzzkill, the drug is not a cure, but it keeps YOUR Restraining Order active.

My 2nd Act officially began when I was declared in clinical complete remission in January 2015. And YOU – Mr. Buzzkill – were not invited to the party.

I live my 2nd Act in complete love and gratitude. Every day is a precious gift to me and I want to pay it forward. I love being here on earth, but I am not afraid to die. And Mr. Buzzkill, YOU need to know that I am not afraid to live.

So I asked myself: "What do I want to be and do when I grow up? What does my 2nd Act look like?"

First of all, I pay it forward with laughter. I never thought I would go from being a university professor and art director to doing stand-up comedy. But there I was on stage, having performed professionally three times so far. And I plan on putting together a routine for cancer patients. Laughing at life is a great distraction from the pain of knowing you have cancer.

During my struggle with YOU, Mr. Buzzkill, I looked for other distractions. My old dog Sir Piss-a-Lot (may he rest in peace) was a great companion and a positive distraction from my cancer treatments and medical tests. Sometimes I think about getting another dog. I think I would name her "Chemo." I want one of those Mexican hairless dogs. After all, hair is over-rated.

Secondly, Mr. Buzzkill, because of my battle with YOU, I push to support others in my 2nd Act. When YOU create chaos and cause others to be frozen by their cancer diagnosis, I become their strong patient advocate. I am one of the founding members of a cancer support group with the focus on living in the here and now. It is called "Living Well," otherwise known as "Not Dead Yet."

Thirdly, because of YOU, Mr. Buzzkill, my voice is louder. I have been invited to speak around the country, sharing my journey of survival with cancer patients, drug sales reps, medical personnel, and caregivers.

Because of the battle that YOU and I have had, I became politically active. I flew to Washington, D.C. to march on Capitol Hill, meet with Congressmen and women, and lobby against YOU with regard to the cost of cancer drugs.

I am the Poster Child for cancer research fundraising. Together with my family and friends at the Leukemia & Lymphoma Society, hundreds of thousands of dollars have been raised in my behalf for cancer research. I share my survival story and the research that saved my life through blogging – *Dr. La Verne's Awesome Adventure: Slaying the Leukemia Dragon.* (www.DrLaVerne.blogspot.com)

Finally, Mr. Buzzkill, YOU cause me to re-examine what brings me joy every day. It is my friends who treat me like I don't have cancer, my husband Carl, my family, and most of all sharing the lives of my 14 grandbabies. It is my art and poetry. It is in those quiet moments that my heart and soul sing for joy. And YOU are nowhere to be found.

Now that I think about it, YOU really didn't steal anything from me. My life has just taken a different path.

By the way, I just had my kitchen cabinets refaced. This is significant. It means I plan on being around to enjoy them. There was a time I wouldn't even buy green bananas. I believe there is still more to my 2nd Act.

So you see, Mr. Buzzkill, – I'm looking at you when I say this – don't mess with MaMa La Verne!

CHAPTER 5

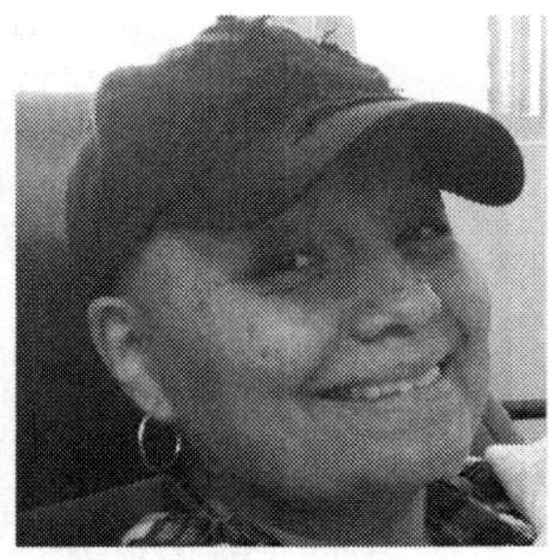

MELINDA MONTOYA

Breast Cancer Survivor

Melinda Montoya, a Las Cruces, NM, native has been blessed with the support of a loving family. She is passionate about inspiring others through her story of recovery and resilience, and motivated to help others through her volunteer work with Cancer Survivors Circle of Strength of Arizona.

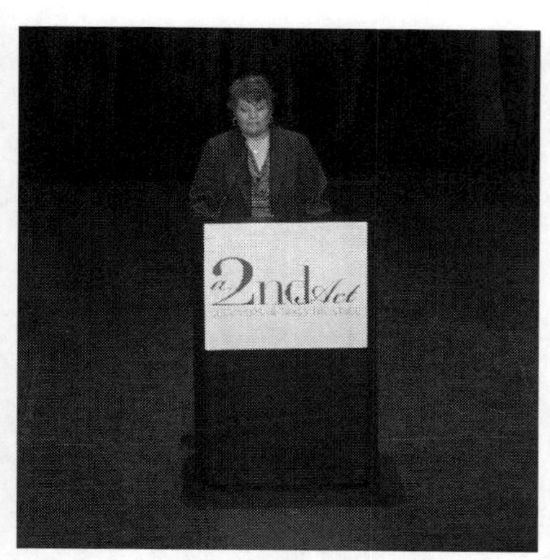

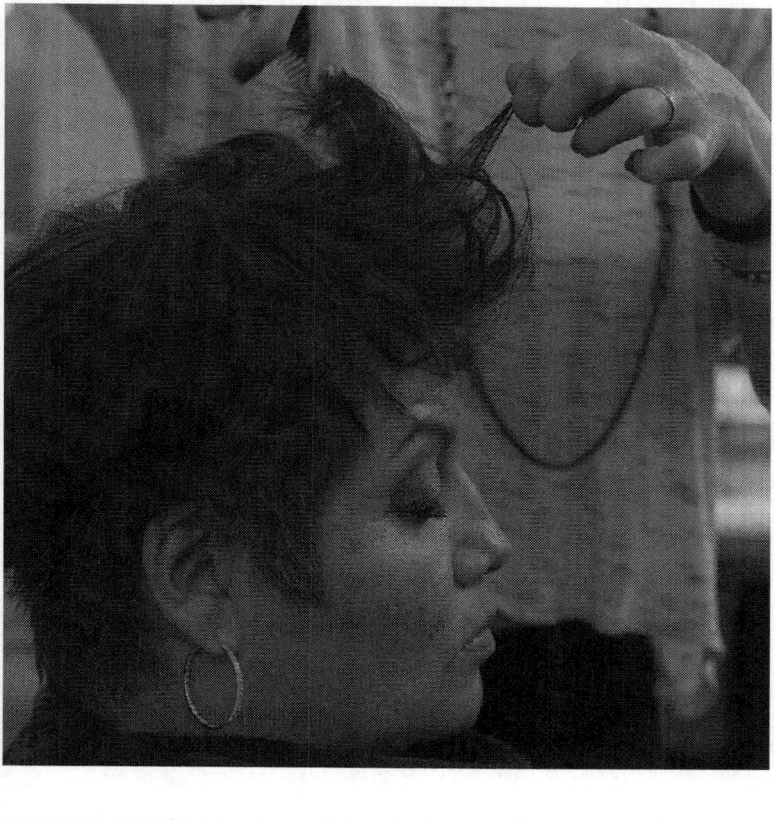

CHAPTER 5: MELINDA MONTOYA

When I went to my very first cancer support group meeting, I didn't really know what to expect. My thoughts were still back at my doctor's office, hearing her say, "You have cancer."

At the end of the meeting we huddled together and the facilitator said, "We're a great team!" I thought to myself, "I don't want to be a part of this so-called team. I never signed up, didn't want to join, and I am not even a big fan of the color pink."

On April 16, 2013, I was diagnosed with breast cancer stage II. Stage II indicates a slightly more advanced form of breast cancer. But thanks to GOD it did not spread anywhere else in my body. I was going to have a tumor removed from my right breast, would need some bit of radiation.

But ensuing results from an MRI and CT scan were not good. I had to make a decision, and scared as I was; I decided to have a double mastectomy.

In going through the journey of being diagnosed with breast cancer, the thoughts and real images of not having any breasts on your body are surreal. I was at a new-comers' meeting at the Cancer Support Community and I met a woman by the name of Judy.

We were there filling out paperwork and being interviewed by the facilitator. Judy had already gone through a double mastectomy but was not able to have the breast reconstruction at the time due to her type of cancer. To my surprise she asked "Would you like to see my scars." I thought, "Seriously?"

At first I was taken back and shocked, realizing that I was going to look like that in a few days. As I listened to her talk, she became so beautiful, almost like a queen of some sort. She spoke with such confidence and grace that I was taken back, and in the end, I saw no scars.

I am reminded that there is nothing wrong with me that I can not give to GOD to be made right. Believe it or not He sees us AS perfect. With Him there are no scars. The scripture in Song of Solomon 4:7, says, "He exclaimed, oh my love how beautiful you are! There is no flaw in you."

I once heard GOD say...."There is no scar, you are beautiful to me. Even in your time of despair and what you see and view as ugly, I have seen you, my child, as beautiful."

Believe me I could not have made up those words. Then it all turned around. My 2nd Act. Now there is no other team or group that I would rather be a part of. I am honored to be in the same room as these women with me up on this stage.

I see things differently and I believe a miracle happened. More like miracles! I truly believe GOD made me stop and realize, "So you're not getting what you asked for, but look at what you have." What I asked for was a phone call, a doctor on the other end saying, "Melinda Montoya, we are so very sorry, we made a mistake, you don't have cancer after all." What did I have when I really looked?

The following.

So many people helped me during my journey. My company, United Cerebral Palsy of Central Arizona, that I am so proud to be a part of gave me strong support. I was anonymously given over 150 hours of paid time off. Someone paid medical bills; someone else paid my rent one month. Judy Gates, the mother of Cody Gates who was one of my students, made t-shirts for me.

My two sisters, Debbie and Minerva, traveled from New Mexico and stayed to care for me. Every morning they would wash me up, schedule my meds, drain my chest tubes, and yes, even wipe my behind.

They weren't always perfect nurses. One of them once asked me to hold the box of bathroom wipes. I started to read the back of the container because I really had nothing better to do. It said, "Works great on boats and automobiles."

She had grabbed the wrong box - they were cleaning wipes, not bathroom wipes. But they put their hearts into caring for me.

Then there was my amazing Nikki who drove me to every appointment, sat with me through every round of chemo, along with her boxer "Trapper." They never left my side. I will never forget when Trapper noticed I was crying.

I had just finished taking a shower and my hair was coming out in clumps. I had my face covered with a towel. I looked up and there he was. He put his head on my lap to comfort me.

Nikki researched books, cooked incredible healthy meals. I became a vegan for four months, and she came up with a new and improved way to lose weight, she called it VEGO!! A combination of being vegan and getting chemo.

The cards, letters of hope and love kept pouring in. Now, I want to help others. I want to bring love and hope to others because of all the changes that occurred within me.

So what's changed? I am doing things I never thought were possible. Things I never could have imagined.

First, my job changed. I was diagnosed with PTSD as a result of my cancer journey. It's not unique; it happens far more than people realize. It became very difficult for me to be a program lead in the special needs classroom where I spent my days.

During one of my dark days, and I had many. The days that fear and questions about my life set in. The day's that I hurt physically, I hurt mentally, and my heart was broken. I asked GOD, "What do I do? I feel so lost, what do I do?"

And I heard back, "What do your kids do?" The kids that I supervised and taught all have special needs. From autism, downs, cerebral palsy, they all have some form of disability.

I thought of the kids that I had taught for over 10 years. I saw them running on the playground, laughing, smiling. They were living! Some of these children have permanent disabilities, but they were still living. I believe they taught me to do the same.

So my company created a new position for me. I am now working on training and becoming an instructor to help staff work better with the members we serve. I was given a new title, you know when my wonderful boss Terry Wideman came on board with us she used the word "Compliance" a whole lot. So much that at our staff meetings I would think "If she says COMPLIANCE one more time, I am going to stick a fork in my eye." The result? My new title is Program COMPLIANCE Specialist!

As a result, I've done and learned so many new things. I am continuing my training for certification as a prevention and support instructor. I teach intervention emergency physical techniques to be used as a last resort in an emergency situation.

I surprised myself because training for this class is physically demanding. It made me smile because I remember when I couldn't even lift my arms, when I cried uncontrollably and I could barely walk.

I'm also a certified Article 9 instructor. I teach newly hired staff and those who need to be re-certified about a law that was established through Department of Economic Security in the late 80's. This law has to do with rights of those with disabilities.

But my 2nd Act is so much more. I am a member of the Circle of Strength Cancer Survivors of Arizona. We volunteer almost every weekend for all types of cancer events. True, getting up at 4:00 or 5:00 on a Saturday morning gets rough, but meeting so many amazing people, the serving and giving back makes it all worth it!

I was also asked to write about my journey with breast cancer for a chapter in a book. It was a dream come true for me. It allowed me to become a published author and to share my stories with so many people. Thank you Peggi Peasly. In today's world, either someone is going through what I went through or someone knows someone else who is going through it. I feel privileged that I have the opportunity to try to touch so many.

Before breast cancer, I thought I was living. But now I have walked the path. I certainly have my scars: I know the feeling of having chemo, the sense of crawling out of your skin. I have lost my hair (and I had a lot of hair – think Lion King on a girl!).

In my 2nd Act, I am aware. I try to live intentionally. The flowers are much more, the sun, moon and stars. I try to live in the present and enjoy each moment.

People are so valuable to me and I realize everyone has a purpose.

Most importantly, this is what I took from my journey. I was reminded that this life is not about me. It is about others, and that is where the meaning is. It is where the blessings lie. GOD has given me a gift and I want to share it freely.

I Made It Rain in the Desert

By Melinda D. Montoya

I don't know how it started
I saw no clouds around,
I was staggering on some dry land
Cracking and crushing the earth below
No rain to be found.

But I kept falling forward,
I felt so alone,
But with God's mercy and grace
I was finding my way home.

I made it rain in the desert
With the tears from my eyes.
My first life was lost,
I had to say goodbye.
It's all for the purpose
of making it rain in the desert.

I will cross paths with you,
We will make it rain together,
You are true beauty to me,
Your love and heartfelt compassion
have embraced me tenderly.

Together we will walk tall
and through it all
Hand-in-hand in the Arizona sun
We will make it rain together,
And find our way home.

I am a survivor.

(Dedicated to my sisters and their amazing 2nd Acts!)

CHAPTER 6

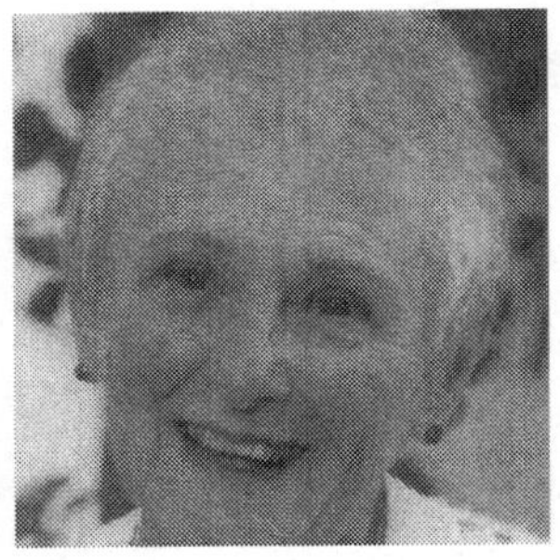

DIANE MILNE

Burkitts Lymphoma Survivor

Diane Milne, a Gilbert resident, is a miracle. She founded Dorothy's Gift, providing Guided Imagery CDs, DVDs and players to cancer patients, both in hospitals and at infusion centers. She also founded and teaches Craft, Create, Heal, fostering healing through creative expression. She is currently working on building a cancer comfort house. And she rocks Zumba!

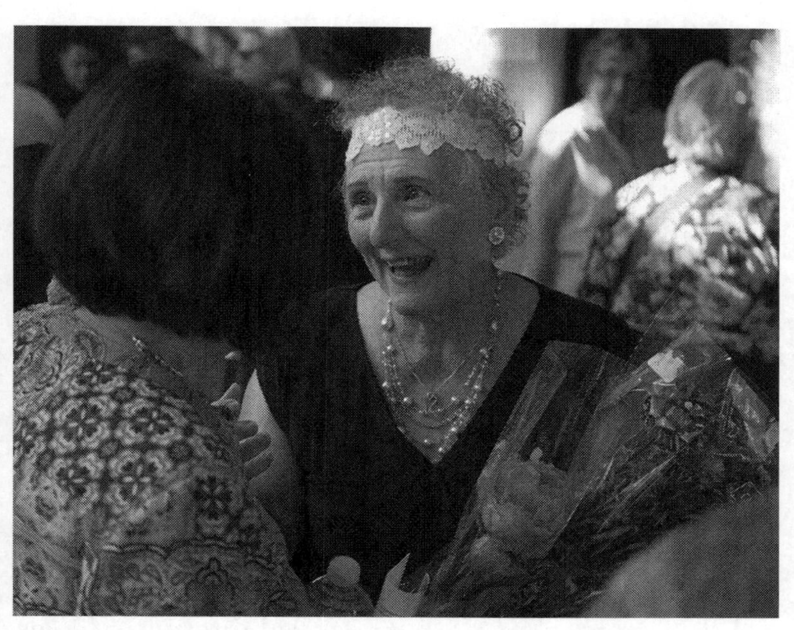

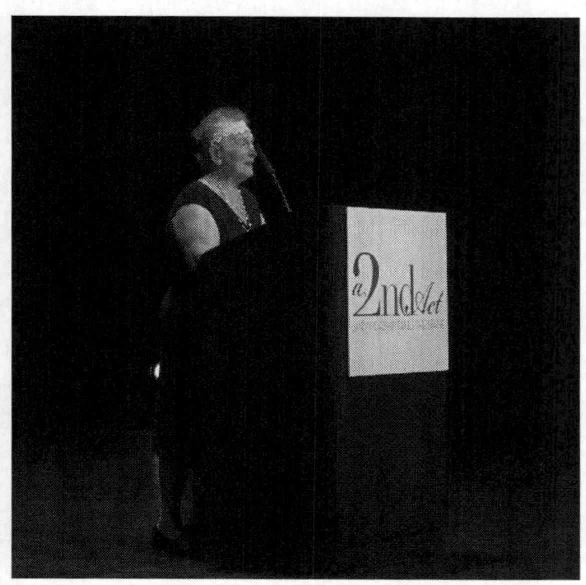

CHAPTER 6: DIANE MILNE

I'm Diane and I'm a miracle. I have one of the rarest and most aggressive cancers on earth. It is a children's cancer that I got at 67 years young. Less than 1% of the world has it. But in my brokenness is blessedness.

I was active, happy, and retired from a 37 year nursing career. My days were filled with Zumba, teaching craft classes at our senior center, and making angel wing handouts for the veterans hospital and cancer patients. My 2nd Act was born after my 1st Act came to an abrupt conclusion on a hot June day in 2014.

I went out to turn on the pool pump before leaving to visit my hospitalized husband. I opened the gate and walked 6 steps when my life changed forever. My heart stopped, I had no breath, no pulse. I knew something critical was happening. I couldn't call out, I had no voice. Frozen somewhere between this world and another I prayed: "God I am dying."

As my hand clenched the fence, the air around me became intensely bright and warm, then only whiteness surrounded me. I saw a figure walking away from me. It was me. I called out, "Wait, wait, I'm still here!" I saw myself turn towards me and smile, and immediately I was filled with peace.

I will never be able to tell you how I made it back into the house or called for help. The next thing I remember is being in the emergency room. At the foot of my bed was a cardiologist I had known for 30 years. There were tears in his eyes. "I don't know how you survived," he said. I had experienced a massive blood clot.

The cause? Hormones secreted by an enormous tumor above and below my diaphragm, extending into my stomach. It had begun to hemorrhage and was inoperable. A bone marrow biopsy revealed that I had Advanced Stage 3 Burkitts Lymphoma, a highly aggressive, highly advanced cancer.

I had inoperable bleeding, deep vein thromboses in both legs, and my right kidney and ureter were already forever crushed by the tumor. All of this was complicated by my now damaged heart. My future narrowed to a few days.

Enter from stage left: my hero and oncologist, Dr. Rohit Sud. He took my hands and in his compassionate kindness explained, "You are not in the literature. But if you will fight, I will fight with you." Our only option was brutal chemotherapy to be done as inpatient over the next six to eight months.

There were times in the middle of the night when I cried, not knowing or believing I would see morning. The winds beat against us, but God has placed within each of us the gift of Hope. Like a little bird holding on to a branch during a storm, we can say, "if you knock me off this limb I'll be OK—God gave me wings". My faith comforted me… God touched me.

During my initial month long hospitalization, the 4th of July arrived. I asked to have my bed wheeled to the sunroom so I could watch the fireworks. I remembered how, as a young nurse on an adolescent cancer unit, we used Guided Imagery. We would have patients visualize cancer cells shrinking or Pac Men gobbling them up.

I began seeing each next beautiful fireworks starburst as a cancer cell exploding and and turning into beautiful proteins my body could use. The next day, I asked for tapes of Guided Imagery but nothing was available. I knew then, this was my purpose, my passion, my vision to help other cancer patients.

I purchased a set online and used them daily. Dr Sud would come in my room and find me with earphones on. I'd tell him, "I'm busy blowing up cancer cells." I danced Zumba down the halls with chemo running, pushing my IV pole with sometimes five pumps across infusing multiple drugs.

I made banners with positive affirmations and hung them all over my room. The doctors and nurses called it the "Happy Cancer Room."

Daily I wore a jaunty flower clipped to a headband because I had no hair. I danced to Pharrell's "Happy," stopping in other patients' rooms, placing the earphones on them, and we sang together.

Curtain up on my 2nd Act!

At a cancer event I met Jude La Cava, a Phoenix

Fox news sports anchor. I introduced myself as usual. "Hi, I'm Diane. I'm a miracle."

I told him about my plans to open a guided imagery library for cancer patients. He told me about his mother who had lost her life to cancer, but had fought hard using guided imagery. He said, "I will help you," and he did.

Through his generosity, and with the help from the Dignity East Valley Foundation, I was able to open Dorothy's Gift at Chandler Hospital last August, named in honor of Jude's mother's courage on her cancer journey. We opened with over 50 CDs and DVDs and personal players.

This February, Dorothy's Gift opened at the Ironwood Cancer and Research Center's Infusion units in Chandler. The program is set to open in Gilbert very soon and plans are underway to open at five additional Infusion Centers. Just recently, we also opened at the two new Comprehensive Cancer Centers in Gilbert and Chandler.

As a cancer advocate and volunteer, I founded and teach "Craft, Create & Heal" for cancer patients at all levels of treatment and their support teams. With help from friends, I also make and take treat bags which get delivered with hand holding, hugs, shared stories and love. Patients share with me because they know I understand like no other.

I have a vision and am currently working with Truth,

Love, Change Foundation to build a cancer comfort house. The plans are already rendered, and I know God will provide the means. After all we only need $2 million and then we can get started.

Above all, I am grateful to my creator for the extra time to cherish each day and bless others on their journey. I encourage you to be as I am—like a little child filled with wonder at the beauty of green grass, the puffy clouds, blue skies, stars twinkling, spectacular sunsets and the tiny flowers growing from cracks in the concrete.

I am grateful to my family and friends for being the wind beneath my wings, so I can fly.

Within each of you are unique gifts that only you can deliver. You have within you the God given power to create a blessed journey for others. Be the stone cast into the still waters. Create a ripple that continues ever outward in growing love.

Live your story, and sing your song, let others dance to your music. And yes… I still do Zumba! Live in expectation for glimpses of angels and heaven, and you will see them. Hold to HOPE, be joy filled and courageous. Remember, today you have met a miracle.

CHAPTER 7

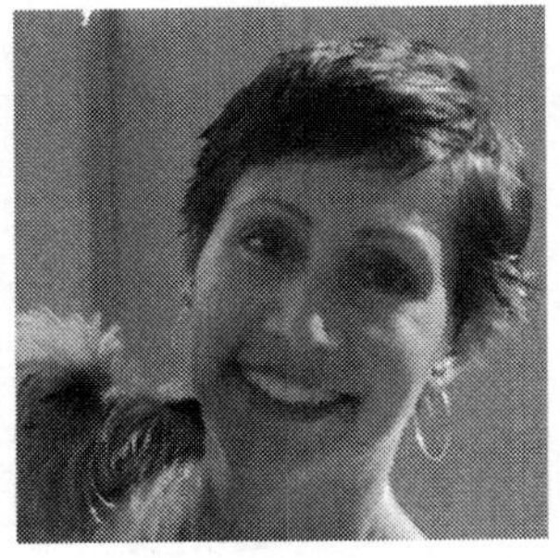

CAT BENDURE

Melanoma and Triple Negative Breast Cancer Survivor

Cat Bendure lives in Phoenix with her husband, and best friend, Ryan, and their three dogs. She's been focused on a journey of self-discovery since receiving her cancer wake-up call. She loves volunteering with Luv of Dogs rescue and is writing her first book.

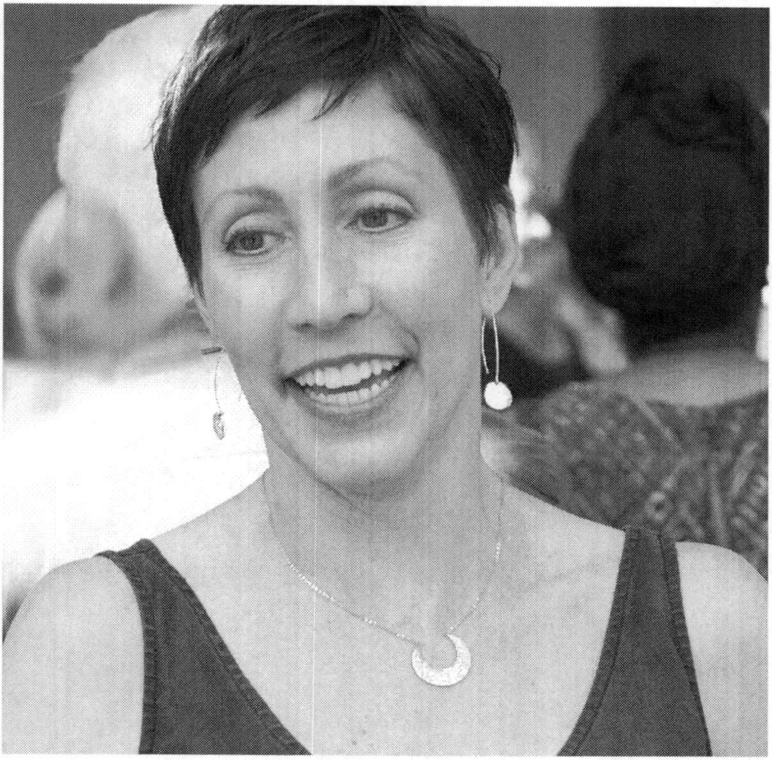

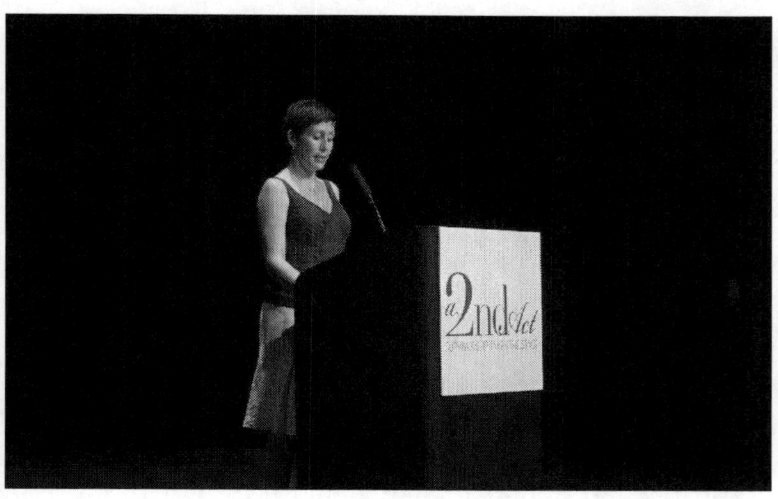

CHAPTER 7: CAT BENDURE

In 2012 I was diagnosed with invasive ductal carcinoma, stage 2b, grade 3, triple negative breast cancer. The tumor was about the size of a golf ball and was in my lymph nodes too. That meant the next 8 months of my life would consist of little more than chemotherapy, surgery and radiation.

I didn't know it then, but that part of my journey, coupled with the years of difficulty that would follow, would become the bedrock upon which I'd build the foundation for the 2nd Act of my life.

I was a successful – although over-stressed – mortgage banker. And while I had tried really hard to work during treatment, I just couldn't do it. I was too sick and too tired and had no ability to think clearly. After I completed treatment, I again tried to pick up my responsibilities, all the things I'd done so well for so long. But try as I might, I couldn't perform the duties that my profession required.

I was no longer sick all the time, but I was exhausted all the time and I wouldn't be able to think clearly for approximately two more years.

I'd worked hard for nearly two decades to achieve the things I had. I was scared and I was angry, but my difficulties were very real and they forced a very real decision. I finally chose to let it all go.

I engaged in activities at the cancer center because I couldn't do much else – yoga, meditation, Chi Ghong,

Tai Chi, and art therapy, you name it, I did it.

And what I found in the quiet calm of these activities were expansive moments – moments that allowed me to begin to let go of old things that no longer served me. And that in turn created the space for new possibilities to develop.

These gifts of time and a slower pace, along with the need to face my own mortality, have given me the opportunity to redesign myself; to remember who I am and why I was born in the first place.

I believe I came to be, with my unique personality, talents, interests and dreams, for a purpose. I've realized that cancer was a gift, a wake-up call and a chance to revive the creative, passionate, intuitive woman I am: the one who'd gotten lost in the hustle of the too-busy life I'd been living. Because when I got lost, so did my dreams.

I've wanted to write books since I was five years old. It was important enough to me that I got a college degree to support that endeavor. But then I chose to listen to the people around me who said I'd never be able to make a living doing it.

I've also always had a passion for working with animals. And I used to do that, before I chose to listen to the same people who again said I'd never make enough money working with animals.

When I revived the woman I'd lost, these dreams

started to feel more like imperatives.

I no longer believe there's no way to make enough money (whatever that is) by doing these things. Gradually, as I've allowed myself to just be, and learned to love and honor the woman I am, I've come to realize that I have these dreams for a reason.

These dreams and abilities are my calling. They're my 2nd Act. And I don't believe we're given the gift of dreams without also being given the ability to achieve them.

That's not to say that I don't ever struggle with health issues and financial issues and all the normal stuff of life. I do.

But what I've found to be a bigger struggle, and this surprised me, is how difficult it can be to choose to do the things you love, and to have the faith that if you follow your dream, work hard, and pour your all in to what you do, that you will succeed.

So I am kind to myself and patient with myself when I falter. I remind myself that it's not a race. And I am very proud to be able to say that I am now pursuing my dreams. I'm writing my first book. In fact, I've been so inspired that I've actually been working on more than one.

My 2nd Act also includes volunteering with Luv of Dogz, a local dog rescue organization. And I've recently begun training dogs again, which I used to do a long time ago. I'm loving it. I'm building my little slice of heaven here on earth, one brick at a time, one day at a time.

I'm choosing to do the things that feed my soul. I take the time to just stop and be quiet, and I allow myself to feel, and to receive the guidance that comes from within when I do this. I listen to my intuition and I've learned to say, "no thank you," when I'm asked to do things that I don't have time for or that just don't feel right for me.

I've also found that I need to remind myself, regularly, that if I wasn't feeling fear or trepidation at the thought of my dream, it wouldn't be BIG enough! I choose to breathe through the fear and uncertainty I feel because I do know that living as my true self, my whole self, even if it sometimes feels like flying without a net, is the stuff dreams are made of.

I am striving every day to live the rest of this life pursuing things that matter to me, even if they matter only to me. I believe that if I do this, I will make a difference in the world.

I know I can have a positive impact on the lives my work will touch. For me, it's the perfect 2nd Act!

CHAPTER 8

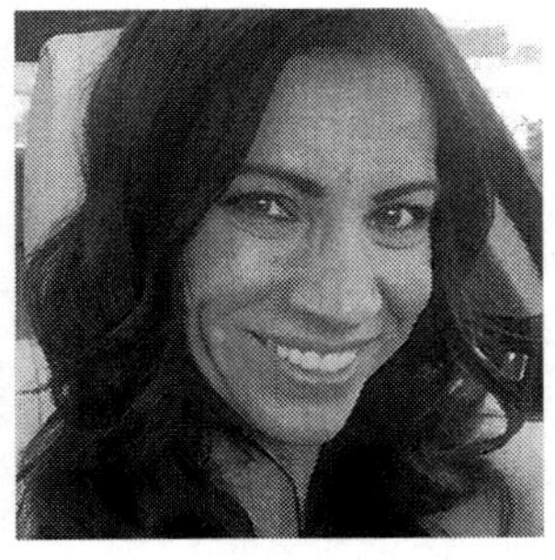

ANGELA DOONAN

Hodgkins Lymphoma and Thyroid Cancer Survivor

Angela Doonan has been a wife and mother for nearly three decades and is a two time cancer survivor who empowers others to fight for their health. A fitness enthusiast known as the "Loco-motivator," her story motivates people online and through national magazines. Her mission is simple: Exercise is powerful medicine!

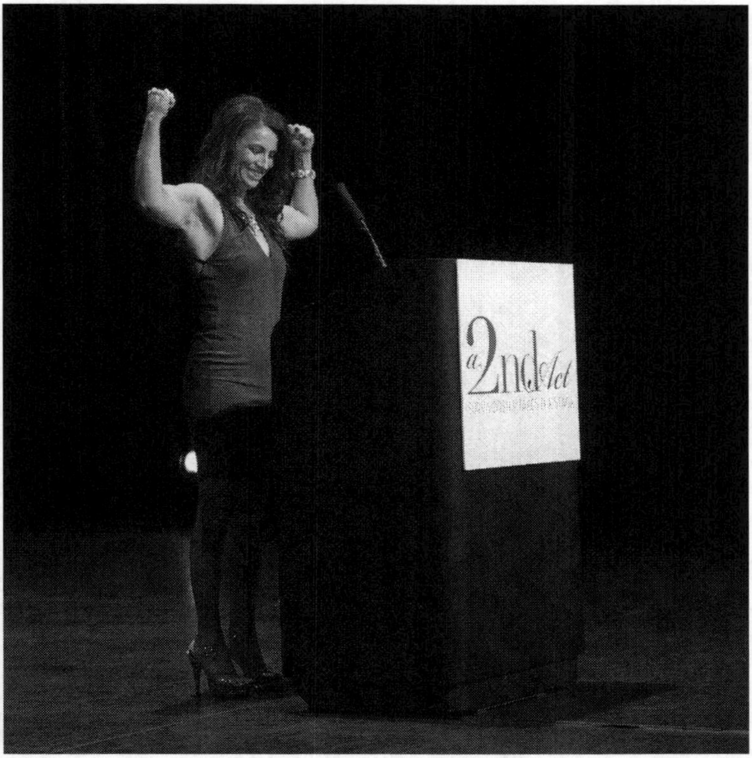

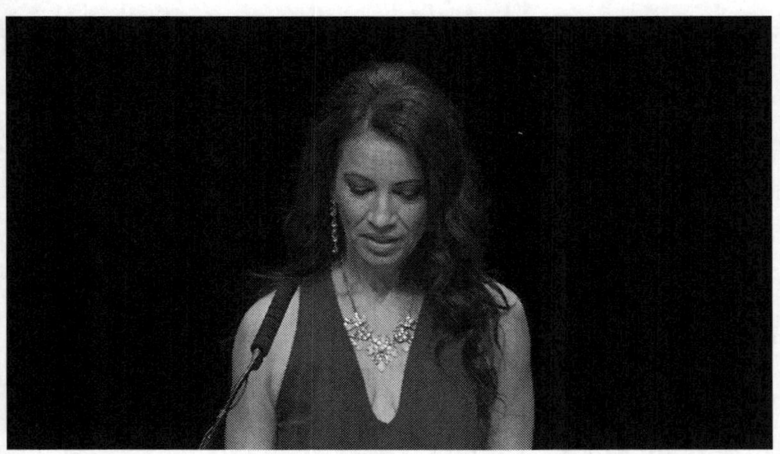

CHAPTER 8: ANGELA DOONAN

Did I ever think I'd be where I am today? Body building? Showcasing health and hope in a bikini to the sick and diseased, to those suffering from the symptoms of obesity?

Did I think as a survivor of Hodgkin's Lymphoma and thyroid cancer that it was even possible to be a poster child for the proven scientific benefits of faithful physical exercise?

Ten years ago, I couldn't have imagined any of those things. My body was left obliterated with the effects of chemotherapy and radiation. I had suffered significant heart and renal failure from all the treatments, as well as the total loss of my thyroid.

Losing my thyroid would cause rapid weight gain leaving me 100 plus pounds over-weight. It didn't take long before I developed all the diseases that come along with obesity: pre-diabetes, high blood pressure, high cholesterol, atherosclerosis and a fatty liver.

But the nail in my emotional coffin was the death of Samantha, my 13-year-old daughter, just eight months prior to my diagnosis with thyroid cancer.

By late 2010, the doctors could no longer assist me in the quality of life I was in such desperate need of! I had given up emotionally. I was ready to just stop fighting for me.

But my husband wasn't. I can still see his outstretched

hand; I can still hear him say, "Let's go for a walk!"

These are truly the moments that define us all as fighters. On those walks around our neighborhood with my husband, I clearly remember feeling awful and barely being able to catch my breath.

I cried a lot, I begged him to slow down. He'd just look back at me and say "Come on, keep going. You've got this!" I hated him at times, but gradually I learned to appreciate his tough love! I kept fighting day after day. I had to learn how to push past all the underlying symptoms of my pain and disease.

I learned to utilize the memory of my daughter, Samantha, who was bound to a wheel-chair her entire life. I would tell myself, "Shut up and walk!" Days turned into months, months turned into years, and those 15 minute walks turned into 10 mile walks!

Did I think those walks were even possible?

Soon I attempted hiking, even though at the beginning I would stop every 15 minutes to catch my breath. But soon what took me an hour and half would eventually only take me 45 minutes!

Did I ever think those hikes were even possible?

Those hikes built up muscles I didn't even know I had! My body started to change out-side and I could feel a change on the inside. I really truly fell in love with physical fitness and never wanted to stop moving.

Did I ever think I would fall in love with exercise?

I had a few set backs including the repair of a subclavian artery that was fully blocked because of radiation damage. I had to spend the next six months fairly bed bound while recovering. And that really sucked!

Who knew how much better I would feel that first hike back on my mountain with proper blood flow? And who knew that an angiogram would reveal that my body had created four new natural bypasses within my heart?

And it all came from me getting my heart rate up daily and fiercely pumping blood throughout my body. Like my husband, my heart was not about to give up on me. Did I think that my faithful stewardship would demonstrate that we were so fearfully and wonderfully made? My body was showcasing the science and redemptive power of physical fitness!

Like many of you, I had a list of "ologists." They understood the power of physical fitness and good nutrition and they soon began to share my story with their patients with the hopes of inspiring them to fight for their health with exercise.

So that brings me back to "Did I ever think I'd be where I am today? Did I ever think this would be my 2nd Act? Or that I'd even have a 2nd Act?"

Motivating tens of thousands with my story being told in some of the most respected national magazines and on television; my doctors sharing my story with the sick; or me on stage in front of all of you; or as a bodybuilder sharing hope in a bikini, not to show OFF but rather to show CASE health and hope.

The answer is, no, I didn't think I'd be where I am today. But the human will to live and fight is so much more powerful than our doubts. And I need you to know the answer is and should be YES!

Now I'm not going to tell you that exercise cures everything; that's absolutely ridiculous!

But I will tell you with absolute confidence that it aids everyone! How can I say this with such confidence? On the days my daughter received regular physical therapy sessions in her wheelchair she slept better.

It wasn't going to make her walk but it certainly aided in her comfort. Again I say, "Exercise aids everyone!" So I am here today with a heart fully determined to fulfill my 2nd Act; to reach the sick and diseased and those suffering from the symptoms of obesity. Why? Because I was once that individual in desperate need of health hope.

My life experiences have left me full of compassion for the suffering and I'm determined to empower them to fight for their health with faithful exercise! My husband dubbed me the "Locomotivator" because I encourage thousands all over the world to fight for their health with exercise.

I'm a living, walking, not-afraid-of-talking testimonial to the power of faithful physical ex-ercise. As a survivor, I'm here to remind you that you are all amazing badasses and that your bodies are fearfully and wonderfully made, inside and out.

I, and the women I shared the stage with, are all so blessed to have 2nd Acts, and to continue to be able to make an impact in the lives of others.

My 2nd Act is simple: to encourage and motivate the masses that exercise is powerful medicine!

CHAPTER 9

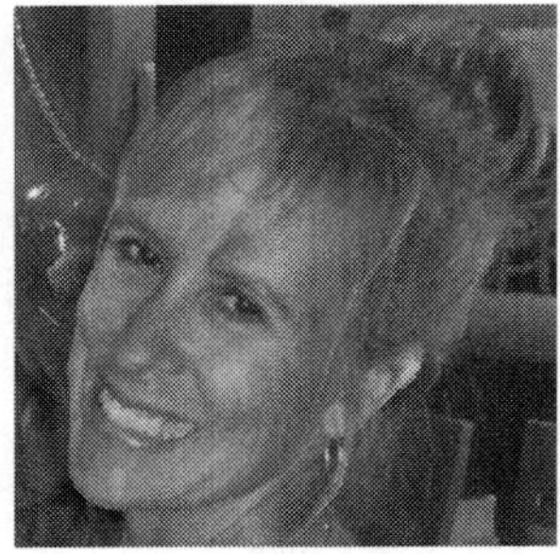

JANELLE HILL

Colon Cancer Survivor

Janelle Hill, a resident of Queen Creek, serves as Chairperson for the Colon Cancer Alliance Central Arizona Chapter. She has been a volunteer with the Chapter for over six years and has served as Chairperson for the past two years. Janelle does Colorectal Cancer advocacy and awareness throughout the state of Arizona and beyond.

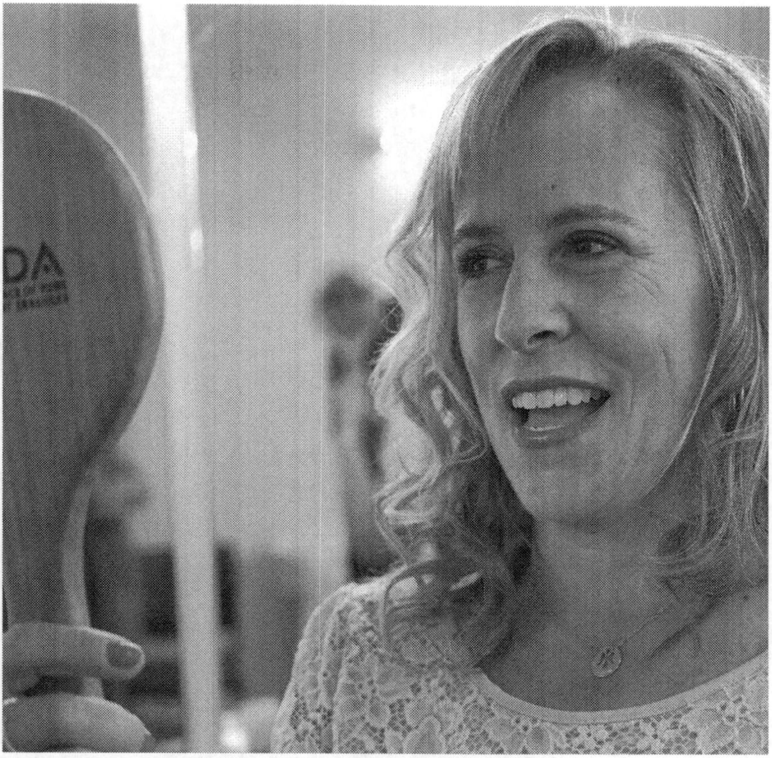

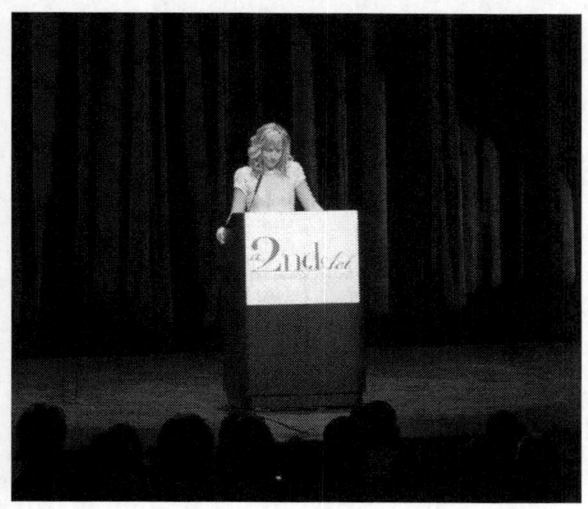

CHAPTER 9: JANELLE HILL

"I cannot believe that I am telling you this but most likely you have colon cancer." Those are the words I heard from my Doctor after I was admitted to the hospital for stomach pain on Wednesday September 15th, 2004. To be honest, I did not even know what colon cancer was. In reality, it was the beginning of my 2nd Act, an act full of poop.

The next thing that I knew, I was being cleaned out in preparation for a colonoscopy. What's a colonoscopy? I had never heard of it. In fact, when I look back on that time I am shocked at how much I did not know about what was happening to me. Not only was everything moving so fast, but much of it was expressed in terms I had never heard of before.

So, lucky me: the colonoscopy could not be fully completed because of the near blockage from the tumor. Surgery was scheduled for the next day.

Approximately eight inches of my colon were removed and while I was in surgery, the test results came back and confirmed that the diagnosis was stage II colon cancer.

Truth is, I had been experiencing stomach pain for a few months before going to the hospital. But I had put off actually seeing a doctor because I was convinced it was the Irritable Bowel Syndrome that I had been diagnosed with four years earlier.

I never fathomed that at 35 years old I would be diagnosed with cancer. My youngest child was just 10 months old. In addition, I was serving as the main care taker for my mom and my dad. Both were under Hospice care, each with an unrelated cancer.

I did not have time to take care of myself. That would have been selfish in light of everything else that was going on in my life. Yup, more poop had been dropped on me.

Three days after my resection surgery I convinced my surgeon to release me from the hospital so I could get home to see my parents one last time. I remember the day quite distinctively ... Monday September 20th. My 36th birthday .... I had just undergone a life-saving surgery. It was the best birthday present I could ever have asked for.

But, I did not receive the same blessing when it came to my mom and dad. My dad passed away the following day from lung cancer and my mom passed away three days later from pancreatic cancer.

It took me five years after my diagnosis to even say the word "cancer." Before that I would always refer to "it" as the "C word." I felt that if I said the word cancer out loud, that would make it real and in my mind possibly make it come back again. Why did I get cancer at 35? Why me? What was I supposed to do now?

Finally I realized that it happened to me for a reason...so I could make a difference in this world. And that is NOT poop.

In January of 2010 I started volunteering with the Colon Cancer Alliance Central AZ Chapter. I knew that I wanted to get involved and start on my new mission, so I Googled colon cancer advocacy on the internet and I found the alliance. It is a non-profit, 501c3 organization based out of Washington DC. But we are fortunate here in Arizona to have a local chapter affiliation.

I attended an open house with the chapter volunteers. It was the first time that I told my story out loud. Of course, I could not keep it together and I broke down in tears.

I looked around at the circle of people surrounding me. Every single person in the room was crying with me. It was at that moment that I knew that I was in the right place. I was hooked. Colorectal Cancer is one of the only preventable cancers and I was going to let anyone and everyone that I could know about it!

I left the open house that day volunteering to be the Chapter Secretary. I began attending health fairs and awareness events with the chapter. I served as Chapter Secretary for two years. Then I got a promotion: I was moved to the Chairperson of The Undy Run/Walk.

The Undy is a 5k Run/Walk held near the State Capitol in downtown Phoenix. This year we will be our 9th year. Because of a partnership with the Arizona Department of Health Services, we designate one half of the net proceeds that we receive locally from the Undy to their screening program for free colonoscopies.

Then two years ago, I got the BIG promotion to Chapter Chairperson.

My role is to communicate with our national office and to keep our board members focused on our mission: to raise awareness through education and screening, to help fund new research, and to provide patient support services for those affected by this devastating disease. Our ultimate goal is to knock colon cancer out of the top three cancer killers.

In the past six years I have helped educate the public about what Colorectal Cancer is, including who is at risk, and when screening is recommended. Per government guidelines, screening is not recommended to begin until the age of 50. But the problem is that we are seeing a rapid increase in those diagnosed under the age of 50. So it makes my "job" that much harder. How do we save our young people?

In general they don't want to talk about their butts, let alone their bowel movements. So how do we get their attention?

Enter "Nolan the Colon," a giant inflatable colon that has been traveling with us throughout the state for 4 years. Nolan even has his own Facebook page! I am not making this up!

Fully blown up, Nolan is 12 feet long, 10 feet high and 10 feet wide. That's a lot of poop! But when people see a giant inflatable colon, they tend to want to check it out. Then I've got 'em.

I can start a conversation and literally walk them through the colon. Inside, we have examples of what normal colon tissue looks like, what a polyp looks like, and what malignant cancer looks like. I know that the greatest barrier people have when it comes to colonoscopies is the" fear of the unknown."

If I can have that one-on-one conversation with that person, especially if it's inside an inflatable colon, I can help to remove those fears and barriers, and "move" them (get it?) to start the conversation about screening with their doctor.

Nolan and I have been to health fairs in Flagstaff and Tucson, and I have attended many events here in the Valley. I've done the South Mountain Climb to Conquer Cancer and the Arizona D-Backs Race Against Cancer. I've also traveled twice to Washington DC to discuss closing an insurance loophole regarding screening.

It is amazing how disinterested people are when it comes to discussing colonoscopies and colon cancer UNTIL they see Nolan AND I inform them that I am a survivor. When colon cancer takes the form of a real person, then they're willing to learn more.

I have no idea how many people I have educated about colon cancer. But I can safely say I rarely go a day without talking to someone about butts and bowel movements. Any place, any time. At Safeway when I am getting groceries or with other parents at my son's football games. In fact, I'm often referred to as the "colon cancer lady".

Even though being diagnosed with colon cancer was the worst thing that has happened in my life, it gave me my life purpose. I'm here to educate the public about a deadly disease with enough accurate information to get them to act, without scaring them. Bottom line, I am here to talk about poop.

In all seriousness, I know that I was "picked" for a reason. I can now see what the footprint that I am going to leave on this earth will look like. What will yours look like?

CHAPTER 10

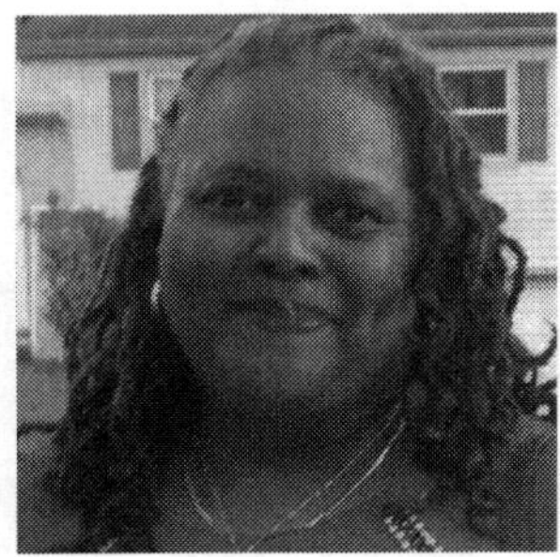

SABRINA A. DOUGLAS

Two-time Breast Cancer Survivor

A Phoenix resident, speaker and community outreach ambassador for Susan G. Komen and the Coalition of Blacks Against Breast Cancer, Sabrina A. Douglas served eight years in the U.S. Army. Mother, and "G-ma," she is a lifeline to many touched by breast cancer. Her cheerleader and caregiver extraordinaire, Al Harris, Jr., has taken this cancer journey with her.

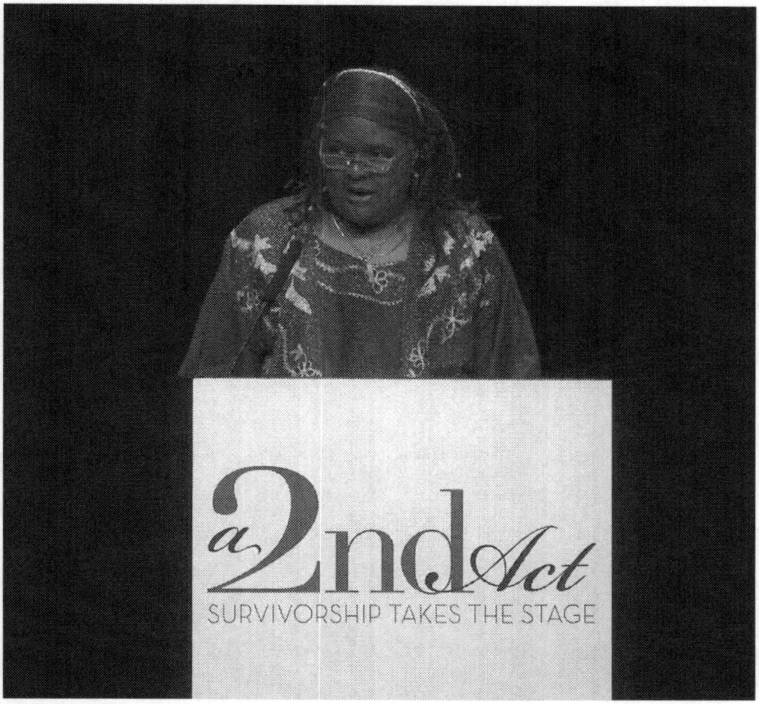

a 2nd Act
SURVIVORSHIP TAKES THE STAGE

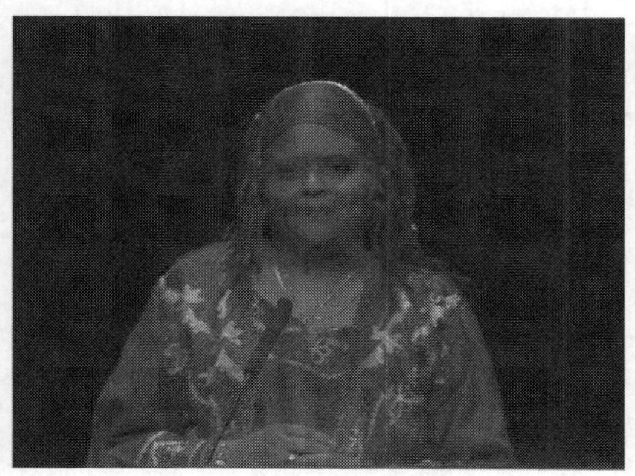

CHAPTER 10: SABRINA A. DOUGLAS

They call me Sabrina "breast cancer" Douglas. It's a direct result of being willing to share my story, of being willing to hold someone's hand, of being willing to listen to the fears and questions that come from finding a lump or being told "You have breast cancer."

I've had a few other names, two that are still with me. Sergeant Douglas (actually Staff Sergeant/E-6), which was earned during eight years in the U.S. Army. When I became a civilian I picked up the name MOTV8HER (Mo-T-V8-Her). She works with many, especially women, as a life coach, trainer and speaker. I'm still called by both names, but the Sergeant and the Motv8Her got lost in the shuffle when the big C came along.

My family has had its share of breast cancer. As a child I lived with a maternal great aunt who had one breast and used "falsies". My mother had Stage III. One of my brothers has even had breast cancer! And, I've had it two times in two years.

In 2008, I found a lump. My journey began with two lumpectomies, the new radiation (twice a day for five-days), and the bonus gift of more than four months of MRSA staph infection.

Then in 2010 I was shocked and saddened when my surgeon told me I needed a mastectomy. My breast cancer was back! My thoughts came fast. Is this metastasized? Is it worse to have it again, so soon? I don't want to die!

Hold on, Sabrina. Get yourself together ... pull up your big girl drawers. Make a plan. The plan was to have a mastectomy and then have the left breast (the one that DIDN'T have breast cancer) removed prophylactically. I made the bold decision that I would not have reconstruction. It took months of working through self-doubt and self-image issues. Now, more than five years later, I still struggle with doubt, but I am learning to love the body I have now!

So then I asked God, "What was I supposed to learn from being a two-time SURVIVOR?" The answers came loud and clear: "Let others know there's life after breast cancer. Even after two times. You'll get to watch your grands grow up. Spoil them. And pay it forward!"

The spoil your grandchildren part was easy! The youngest of my two granddaughters was born in 2009, between my first and second bouts of breast cancer. Looking into her eyes gave me a desperate will to live! She was the fifth of five grandchildren from my son... two girls and three boys. My daughter has given me three boys, the newest was born in January 2016. I recently traveled to Brooklyn, NY, to hold him. It is my ritual to hold each of my grands as soon as possible. To sing a song of blessing, pray for the baby, connect the voice they've heard in utero with a person and rock them to sleep while singing "This Little Light of Mine." A true 2nd Act is being a grandparent!

Having grands across a span of ages ... newborn, toddler, elementary schoolers, junior high, and high school … gives me glimpses into a child's life in 2016. They are my tech team. My 'carry this, get me that' team.

One has been my team captain since he was five and he just turned 13. Damien's in charge of organizing family and friends for breast cancer activities. He's also in charge of all things pink. He wears pink laces, shirts, and caps. Don't challenge him. If you ask, he'll say, "It's for my Grandma" in a terse manner.

They all have assisted in my volunteer efforts. Some have spoken to other kids whose grandmothers have breast cancer. Anastacia, the littlest Princess, knows many of the facts and believes it is her right to attend all events. She was raised on a mat behind many of my volunteer vendor tables.

Volunteering has also been easy. Through my research for my treatment, I learned that my community has some disturbing statistics. African American women have the lowest survival rate of all women with breast cancer diagnoses. Women delay reporting a lump. My own mother waited eight months before she told us about hers. And some women are more concerned about losing their hair than living. I can't make this up!

Enter Susan G. Komen and the Coalition of Blacks Against Breast Cancer (CBBC-AZ). These groups trained me to be an Ambassador to do community outreach. I became armed with my story of survivorship, and their training and educational materials. Volunteer opportunities were plentiful. And my 2nd Act really took off.

This community work led me to become an AmeriCorps Liaison, facilitating workshops on Chronic Disease Self-Management. I've been honored by TV stations, churches and other organizations.

I even received the 2013 Joyce Gooding "Spirit of Komen" award for volunteering.

It's nice to receive awards and accolades. However, I volunteer because I don't want my 7-year-old granddaughter to hear the words "You have breast cancer." I volunteer because African-Americans are dying at higher rates, with some of the most aggressive and late stage forms of breast cancer. I volunteer because I know there is life after breast cancer.

Surviving breast cancer twice has given me another chance to focus on grandchildren, travel, and Al, the love of my life. Surviving breast cancer twice has made volunteering a way of life for me. A way to pay it forward ... my 2nd Act.

CHAPTER 11

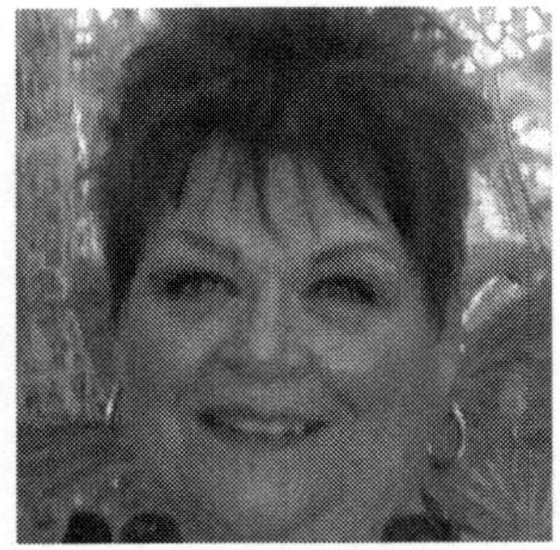

ALLISON SANDERS

Breast Cancer Survivor

Allison Sanders lives in Phoenix and was diagnosed with Stage IV breast cancer in early 2005. Given three to six months to live, Allison hasn't slowed down since. She is the co-founder of Open Wings of H.O.P.E. and the co-founder of Cancer Survivors Circle of Strength of Arizona. Allison understands the impact of cancer on the lives of others and fulfills her life passion to bring hope and strength to them.

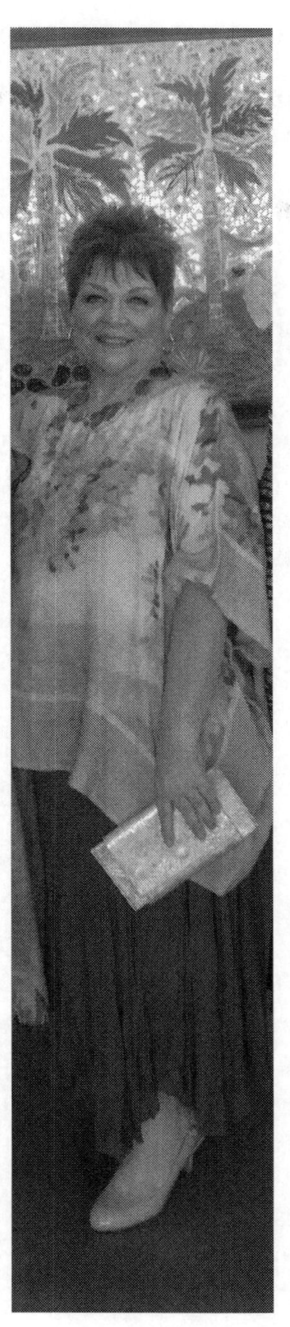

CHAPTER 11: ALLISON SANDERS

When I was preparing my story, I was told I'd only have five minutes to share it. I can't even say hello in five minutes, but I'll try my best!

My first act was all about being a single mother and working for corporate America. I was successful at both and am now the proud mother of a grown son who contributes in a positive way to society. With the help of mentors along the way, I developed many skills working in finance, human resources and leadership training. One of the many skills I learned were interpersonal skills. I love serving others and seeing the light in someone's eyes when they "get it." You know that gleam of "oh, I can do this!" I love that.

In 2005, I was diagnosed with stage IV breast cancer and given about three months to live. Now if I can't say hello in five minutes, I sure can't say goodbye in three months! The timing was not good for me: my son was in college, I had a job I loved, and I was doing well financially. I was too busy for cancer. But as you all know, sometimes God has different plans.

As I stand here today, nine years later and still in treatment. But I want you to know I am pursuing my 2nd Act. I believe my true life purpose is to provide hope to others. HOPE for me is Healing, Optimism, and Personal Empowerment. I am a partner in a small business, called Open Wings of H.O.P.E. With the help of my awesome caregiver and best friend, Teresa Scott, we turned this crazy business of cancer into a cancer survivors manual. It provides newly diagnosed patients and their caregivers a tool to navigate their own personal journey of wellness.

The manual is called the "Survivor Success System" and contains tabbed sections for the different areas of treatment, including calendars, medication charts, physician logs, lab reports, surgery logs and resources. We encourage patients to spend their time getting well, not researching ways to manage the journey. Providing resources also helps them to find available social and financial programs.

Other aspects of our organization are patient advocacy and specialized Life Coaching for those touched by cancer. I believe the answer for healing and discovering your purpose is already within you. My job is to help you discover it.

Since we had no financial backing, I started marketing the manual through volunteering at other non-profit cancer related organizations. One purchased 100 books from me and asked me to run a social group for them once a month. I tend to give more away than I actually sell, but I don't mind. The main purpose is to help others.

I am also a founding member and sit on the board of Phoenix-based Arizona Cancer Survivors Circle of Strength. We are a not-for-profit group of volunteers, touched by cancer, that provides service to individuals, families and other cancer-related organizations that may benefit from our experiences. We provide a mentorship program, a listening ear, an opportunity to belong to a community, and resources for others in their own journey. In addition, we provide affiliate partners with volunteers for events, health fairs and programs. We've found that those touched by cancer want to give back in a meaningful way. And isn't that what a 2nd Act is all about?

Additionally, I recently was asked to be the Board Chairperson of Organizational Development for Send Me on Vacation. Send Me on Vacation is a non-profit that sends survivors on a vacation as the first step to emotionally healing. We partner with corporate organizations, providing them with a cancer tool box that includes resources and training for both managers and employees who are working with diagnosed staff members.

I don't have to tell you that surviving is much more than just beating cancer. It is a mind, body, and spirit experience that affects relationships, finances, health, social and mental aspects of life. Knowledge and H.O.P.E. (remember, Healing Optimism and Personal Empowerment) help to eradicate fear and depression, and create a smoother road to healing.

I had a dream and was told to share this with each of you: "Your time as a caterpillar has expired, and your wings are ready! The sound of HOPE is our wings learning to fly. So take flight.

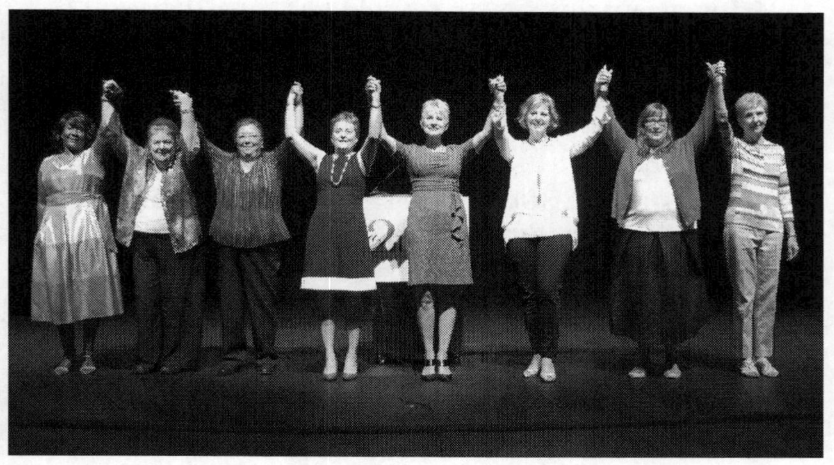

Tucson cast members from left to right:
LaNita Price, Karen Conway, Isabelle Barbour, Susan Kinkade, Judy Pearson, Sara Moore, Lisa Reynolds, Ginny Williams

TUCSON

In the shadows of the Santa Catalina mountains, these women trudged through the darkest hours of cancer. But the disease did not defeat them. Rather it touched their lives in ways they never might have imagined, giving them a new appreciation for every sunrise, and making them stronger and more dedicated in their 2nd Acts.

Sunday, November 13, 2016, 2:00 p.m
Berger Center for the Performing Arts, Tucson, AZ

This performance was made possible by the generosity of Radiation Ltd., Printex, KVOA and MIXfm.

Love to Mrs. Grant, Emcee
MIXfm Morning Mix

CHAPTER 12

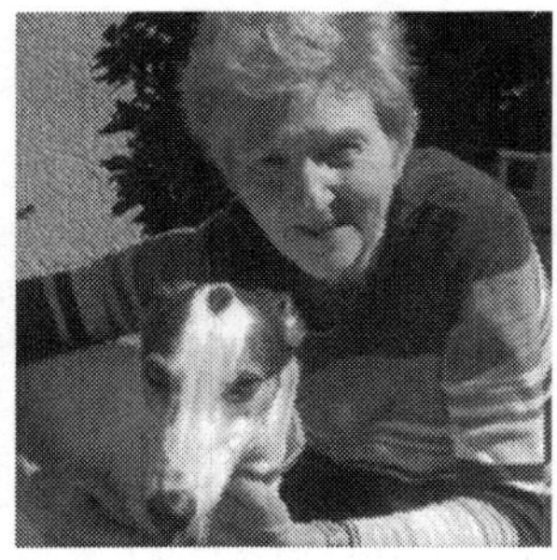

GINNY WILLIAMS

Breast Cancer Survivor

Ginny lived in a coal-mining town in northeastern Pennsylvania until college. There, she earned a B.S., an M.Ed. and an Ed.D degree all in support of her teaching career. She retired from education in 2006 and moved to Arizona, where she works with Southern Arizona Greyhound Adoption. Learn more at www.sagreyhoundadoption.org.

The day of my needle biopsy was the day that I decided that I was going to beat cancer rather than the other way around. There was just no way that cancer was going to take over my life. So, I did what I had planned for that day.

I went to the vet's to pick up (and I mean that literally) a newly spayed greyhound, lifted her into the back of an SUV and took her to her foster home.

And then, two days after my lumpectomy a few weeks later, I did a six mile walk. Normally, I would have taken a hike instead, but I thought that might have been too much, too soon. As it was, my walk was a big mistake.

I bruised so badly that it actually scared me. So, I called my surgeon immediately, and she told me to come right in. The first thing she said to me was: "What have you done?" When I told her, she said that the word "walk" in the post-op instructions meant just around the block – not six miles. OOPS!

So, I went back to doing what I've been doing for almost 20 years – taking care of greyhounds that have just gotten off the track. I'd clean their kennels, feed them and best of all, play with them.

As soon as the dogs would come into our intake kennel, we'd de-tick and de-flea them and give them baths. You just can't imagine how they would respond! Sometimes it was almost as though they went into sleep mode they were so relaxed. At other times they'd respond with a sudden burst of energy and pure joy.

I was just so delighted to be part of their transformation and the beginning of their new lives. For me, it was the best cancer support ever! And I realized then that the rescued greyhounds were a lot like cancer survivors. They, too, had to endure some harsh treatment just as cancer patients suffer through chemo and radiation.

But, at the end of it all, we both have a new appreciation for life. It's a joie de vivre that we have in common and an honor for me to help them begin their 2nd Acts of life.

As you've most likely surmised by now, I also had a pet greyhound at home. His name was Lincoln, and he was truly "my dog." Initially, like many of us survivors, I had a difficult time accepting my diagnosis, so I was often awake at night. But, if I was up so too was Lincoln.

He'd sit beside me and look at me with his doe-like eyes. if I went to take a shower, he'd be lying just outside the bathroom door – all 87 pounds of him! While I lost Lincoln soon after I began chemo, I will never forget him or the love and concern that he had for me.

Because hiking has always been therapy for me, I hit the trails again while in chemo. I began slowly with shorter hikes as I didn't have the same energy level that I once did. It was on one of those hikes when a gal in my hiking group turned to me and said, "You know, you look a lot better than I thought you would." I took that as a compliment because I was even paler then than I am right now!

When I finished treatment and got back some of my energy, I was off on hiking trips that took me to Alaska, Utah and New Mexico. A few weeks ago, I was in Colorado, hiking in snow at 12,500 feet. And, I can't wait to go again!

Until then, though, I'll continue helping newly arrived greyhounds transition to life as someone's pet.
And, even though it's not a mission that is new to me, it means more to me now than ever before. It affords me the opportunity to give back to a breed that has given me so much during this time in my life.

As I look back now, I laugh about some of the things that have happened – my misunderstanding of my surgeon's use of the word "walk" and the left-handed compliment of a fellow hiker. And then there was the trip to the dentist in Nogales, Mexico.

As I was coming through customs, I handed an officious-looking border patrol officer my open passport. He looked at my picture, at me, and then back at my picture once again. Obviously, that pre-cancer picture didn't look much like the person standing before him. I finally said, "That picture was taken before chemo when I had a lot more hair." He softened, smiled and said, "You're a survivor. Good for you."

I think that if that same border patrol officer were here today he'd say, "You're all survivors. Good for you!"

CHAPTER 13

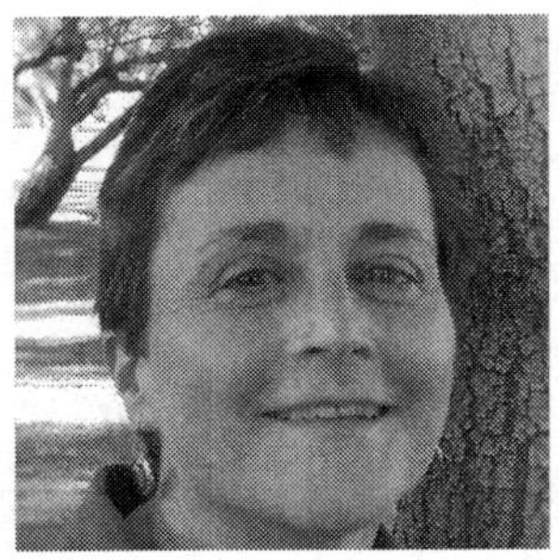

SUSAN KINKADE

Leukemia Cancer Survivor

Susan is a wife, mother, emergency nurse and cancer warrior. She volunteers for the "Be The Match" bone marrow program, as well as with the American Cancer Society Relay for Life. She speaks to nursing and medical students about her experience on the other side of the hospital bed. Learn more about bone marrow donation at www.bethematch.org.

Close your eyes for a minute. Imagine yourself as an emergency nurse who has helped people in their darkest hour for over 30 years. Imagine you haven't been to your doctor for ages because, well, you're a nurse and you know what's going on with your health.

Imagine you went in for some blood work prior to an elective surgery but only because it was required. Imagine waking up after a well-deserved nap on a Friday afternoon and hearing a message on your voice mail from your doctor saying, "If you are still my patient you need to make an appointment right away because you have some abnormal lab work that we need to talk about!"

My Monday morning appointment couldn't come soon enough. In one short conversation I heard three words that changed my life — you have leukemia. Chemotherapy and radiation would treat it, but a bone marrow transplant was my only hope for a complete cure.

Early on, I wanted to keep my diagnosis private. I felt that if I admitted I was sick, I'd have people feeling sorry for me. I didn't want to go to a support group where I was afraid I'd see hopeless people. I struggled with my choice, but everything changed the day I made the decision to go public.

They say it takes a village to walk with you down the cancer road. I found it takes many villages.

I had my family village, my work village, my community village and my church village. Everyone intertwined to support me and my family and carry me in my weak moments.

I met people I never would have met otherwise. I've become closer than ever before to others.

My detour through the valley of leukemia was certainly not all rainbows and roses. Was I scared? Absolutely! I needed stem cells from bone marrow to survive! Being a bone marrow donor is a huge commitment.

The only thing that scared me more than the diagnosis was the thought that my three brothers who live out of state wouldn't agree to bone marrow donor testing. Or if they did, none would be a match. Fortunately, they all agreed and one WAS a perfect match. It's times like this when you really find out how important family is.

Did I go through dark times? Most definitely! I embraced and acknowledged the bad times and chose to move on and celebrate the good things that came my way. A few symbolic items have helped carry me through my journey and will always remain close to me.

When I went in the hospital for my transplant, I asked my husband to find a special rock that I could hold to remind me of him. He has been my true rock and fortress from day one. That rock sits on my desk at work to remind me of how far I've come and the strength and love that he has given me.

As I was walking out the doors of the hospital on discharge day, on my way to a new life, the social worker slipped a small key into my hand. She said, "You earned this." The key has the word "strength" written on it. It took me a while to understand the symbolism of that simple word. Now I do: that key symbolizes the key to life after leukemia. It was up to me to open the door to that new life and begin my 2nd Act.

One of the most important lessons I learned on my journey was patience—with myself, my family and my health care team.

In the early days after my transplant, I was physically weak but mentally strong. I would set small goals for myself like walking to the end of the block or going to church.

As my leash at the cancer center became a little longer, I gained strength and started doing hikes and planning little trips. I continued trying to define what my new normal and my 2nd Act would be.

Six months after my transplant, I got to travel to Oklahoma for my son's graduation from basic training.
I felt like I was on the vacation of a lifetime. I was doing what normal people do!

One year after my diagnosis, I was given clearance to return to work, as long as I didn't have direct patient contact.

The bedside nurse in me really struggled with that but I was able to define "nurse" in a different way. As a trauma outreach coordinator, I transitioned from being an ER nurse to being in the community teaching injury prevention.

On my one year transplant anniversary, I felt like I had conquered the world. I wanted affirmation that I was alive and well. How did I celebrate? I went sky diving! Reaching out and touching the sky was an amazing moment, although probably not the smartest thing to do for someone who has no platelets!

From way up there in the sky, I could feel myself heading back to life's main road and knew that I wanted to spread the message that there is life after cancer. That would be my 2nd Act.

Being on the other side of the hospital bed gave me a whole new perspective of what a patient goes through. Using my experience, I speak to nursing and medical students giving them a view they wouldn't typically get in school.

I also speak to bone marrow transplant patients. They hear about the whole transplant process from their health care team, but sharing my journey gives them encouragement. I give them a "Walk to Wellness" packet that has a pedometer and journal in it.

Hearing that attitude and exercise play a huge part in their recovery is good medicine, and helps them see that while the road is long, there is light at the end of the tunnel.

People have asked me, "At what point do you start counting how long you've survived? My survival started the day I received my diagnosis. It was when I made the affirmation to fight and go where this detour in my life's journey would lead me.

Early on, my doctor and I made a pact that I wouldn't look at research that showed life expectancy after my type of cancer. I have kept that promise. To this day, I don't know how long I'm expected to live.

But to be fair, who among us really does? I feel like each of us is unique and will travel our own journey, regardless of the statistics. I'm not just surviving – I'm thriving! I have made the choice to live every day like it matters.

I have to say that while skydiving was on my bucket list, leukemia certainly wasn't! But as a result of my disease, I have a new passion for life and can't wait to see what the future holds.

Embrace your journey and take each day a step at a time. Let yourself be open to the help of those around you. Celebrate the little things. Live YOUR life like it matters!

CHAPTER 14

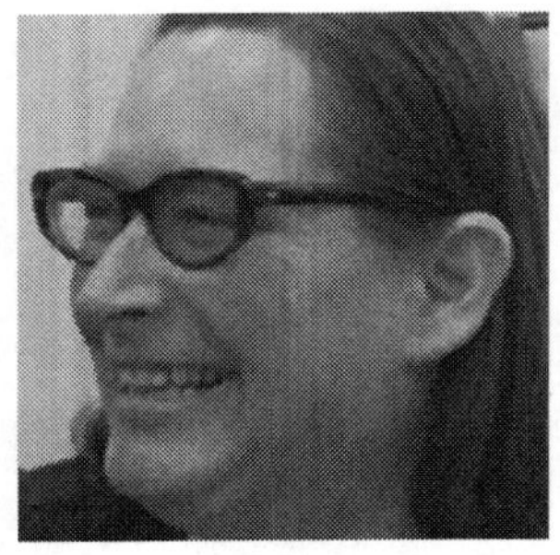

LISA REYNOLDS

Childhood Thyroid Cancer Survivor

Lisa, a resident of Tucson, has been a patient navigator for the American Cancer Society for the past six years. She is an advocate for the American Cancer Society's Cancer Action Network and advocates for more funding for cancer research. She also participates in Relay For Life. Learn more at www.cancer.org

It was 1981. I was 8 and my family was on the way down to Mexico to go sailing. My brother and I were in the back seat doing what siblings do: having an argument.

He said, "You're ugly." So I, of course, responded the same. Then he said, "Well, you have a lump in your neck." And I of course said, "Well, you have a lump in your neck." My mom turned around quickly and said, "Where?" My brother pointed and said, "Right there." And I pointed at him and said, "Yeah, right there."

That was the day I found out boys have Adam's apples and girls don't. In fact, girls aren't supposed to have lumps in their necks at all.

My mom called my doctor when we got home from our trip. His advice was not to worry about the lump' to "just wait and see what happens."

Luckily, my mother didn't listen. She took me to her ear, nose, and throat doctor. The next thing I knew, I was seeing a pediatric surgeon, and a lumpectomy was scheduled.

Following my lumpectomy, I was only able to eat broth and jello. Doctors had finally promised me a milkshake, but before it arrived, we got the news. Thyroid cancer. My mother fainted. I didn't know what cancer was, and I wondered if it meant I wasn't getting my milkshake. And I didn't get one.

Instead, I got scheduled for a total thyroidectomy to be performed a few days later. The cancer was in both sides of my thyroid and had spread to my windpipe. So … it would be surgery and the protocol of the day: a large dose of radioactive iodine.

I had always felt a little bit like an outcast as a child. Getting thyroid cancer at a young age certainly solidified that. It was not a normal childhood cancer. I didn't have normal childhood treatment, and I wasn't in the childhood oncology unit for treatment.

I was in nuclear medicine, the bomb shelter of the hospital. My treatment came in a lead container that no one was supposed to go near. There was a tiny bottle inside that they squirted water in and I drank. Seemed safe.

Once I was able, I went back to school. But having just gone through surgery for cancer, no one would sit by me. Some of the kids were afraid they might catch cancer, too.

Others asked if I smoked. About this time, there was a big anti-smoking campaign going on. As kids, we didn't understand the difference between lung cancer and any other kind, so they all just assumed I was puffing away during recess.

Over the next two years, my cancer was controlled. But then we got word that it had spread to my lungs and my lymph nodes.

In scans, the spots on my lungs looked like lights on a Christmas tree. Decisions had to be made. After some research on my doctor's part. Despite my age, I was now 10, he recommended I receive the maximum adult dose of radioactive iodine.

Because I gave off radioactivity, I was in a hospital isolation unit, with a sign on my door that said, "Caution. Radiation." I was the radiation!

They taped a safety line around my bed, indicating how far back people had to stay to not be exposed. Every few hours, a team would come in with a Geiger counter to test me, and as my radioactivity diminished, they'd move the tape back.

My dad was excited about all of this. Because of emitting so much radioactivity, he figured he wouldn't have to put up Christmas lights up that year. They could just put me on the roof and Santa would find his way.

I was in fifth grade when I was finally declared in remission. And I guess that's the moment my 2nd Act began. I wanted to volunteer as much as I was able given my age. I mostly raised money for the American Cancer Society and the Arizona Cancer Center. But I often felt like a fish out of water.

By the time I turned 16, I had never met another child who had cancer. When I would tell people that I had had cancer, they would ask, "Oh, leukemia?" I would tell them no and they would either lose interest or ask, "Did you lose your hair?" Again I would say no and usually received a look suggesting maybe I didn't really have cancer.

When I first started seeing childhood cancer events, I didn't go. I didn't fit in. Even when I offered to volunteer with other kids who had cancer, they put me with the siblings of cancer patients. Only the kids with normal childhood cancer could relate to current patients. It was assumed I couldn't.

So I volunteered at Arizona Camp Sunrise Sidekicks, a camp for brothers and sisters of kids with cancer. The upside of this was that I learned what it must have been like for my brother when I had gone through treatment.

I was able to do that for five years, until migraines caused me to stop. There's a lot of physical fallout when you don't have a thyroid: rapid heart rate, depression, and migraines as well.

Having gone through two diagnoses, surgeries and hospitalizations, and of course, my "glow" juice treatment (radioactive iodine), I had decided at a young age that I was going to be the one to cure cancer. But my brain wasn't on board.

So, I decided to advocate for money to fund those whose brains were on board! That is when I joined the American Cancer Society Cancer Action Network. I have been to both the State Capitol and Washington D.C. to lobby for increased funding for cancer research.

I continued volunteering at different places and then was lucky enough to be hired by the Ronald McDonald House as a weekend manager.

Then six years ago, my 2nd Act dream came true. A job with the American Cancer Society! Now, I work as a patient navigator, helping patients find the resources they need to get their treatment.

I am so glad to do what I do, but I never feel like I've done enough. There aren't support groups for adults of unusual childhood cancers and we often don't feel as though we fit in to the adult cancer survivor world.

Even the medical world doesn't know how to deal with me. A doctor once called to tell me my tumor marker was high. He didn't know what that meant. I did. It meant I had cancer again.

More blood tests and and a chest x-ray, where the technician asked why I was having a chest x-ray. I told her I had had metastatic thyroid cancer as a child and they thought it had come back. Her response: "Are they sure it was cancer?"

I remembered my two surgeries and multiple radioactive iodine treatments, and replied, "They seemed pretty sure."

I want to help change that. I want to see a day where there are no more children being diagnosed with cancer. And if they are, I want to see them have fewer long-term effects, something I'm so very familiar with.

Many childhood cancer survivors can not have children. In fact, I was told I could not have children. Luckily, this was another time in my life that a doctor was wrong. My 10-year-old son is right here in the audience as proof!

So, the fight goes on and my work goes on. I hope this view from another perspective, a voice from another kind of cancer survivor, will also help you understand my passion … my drive … my 2nd Act!

CHAPTER 15

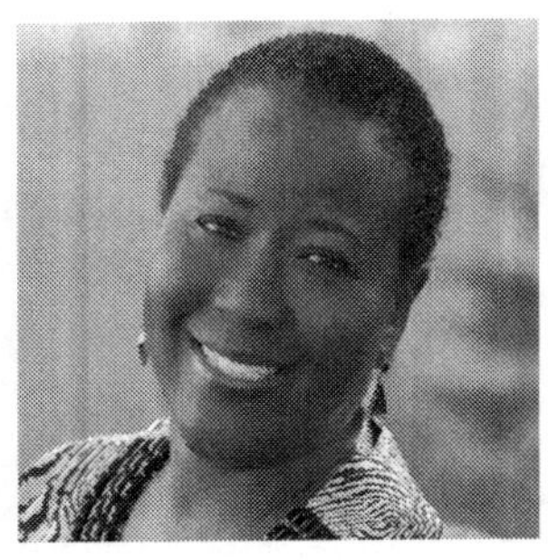

LANITA PRICE

Breast Cancer Survivor

LaNita, a native of Florida, retired from the Air Force in May 2007 and moved to Tucson with her husband Vaughn. They have one daughter and two grandchildren. She is a graduate of Park University with a BS in Social Psychology and a Masters in Addiction Counseling from Grand Canyon University. LaNita has worked in the counseling field and is a licensed minister. She uses her licensure and degrees to help provide life coaching through Healing Hearts Ministries.

CHAPTER 15: LANITA PRICE

What do you do when your slip is hanging?

Funny question I know. But I grew up in Florida and my elders used that saying when someone appeared to have it all together. And then something happened they did not want the world to see.

That was me!

I had been single and celibate for 11 and a half years until I met my now husband. I dressed nice, smelled nice. I had conquered the Air Force and retired as a single mom. I had a nice vehicle, good friends and people labeled me as a good friend and person. I had all the external things that gave me the image I thought I wanted to convey.

Then, in November 2012, the storm came. The wind blew and the ME I had known and loved would change forever and not by choice. Suddenly and without warning, MY slip was about to hang.

I found myself between a rock and hard place when the doctor called me in for my mammogram results. Oddly enough she asked me, "What do you think your results are?"

I said, "Well it can't be good, since they would not give them to me over the phone." She stated that her normal protocol is to have the patient come in and talk with her no matter what the results were.

She then looked me in the eyes and said, "I'm sorry but you have breast cancer Stage II and the surgeons want to operate as soon as possible."

I remember how the tears streamed down my face. On the inside I kept asking, "Me? Are they sure? Me?" The doctor hugged me tightly and told me it would be alright and someone would be contacting me soon to schedule surgery.

As I walked out in the hot Arizona sun, my thoughts and heart went immediately to my husband, Vaughn. We'd only been married five years at this point. He was a widower, whose first wife of 13 years, Yolanda, had died in 2004 due to complications from ovarian cancer treatment.

I never once thought of death, but two big balloons of concern floated into my mind.

First, not only did my husband have to go through his first wife's cancer treatment and death, but now his second wife had cancer too.

And secondly, how was my body going to change? Would I lose my hair? One or both of my breasts? Would nausea, weight loss, loss of energy and who knows what else plague me?

And what would other people think? You know when the big "C" word is said to someone, whether to the patient or anyone else hearing it, more often than not people immediately assign a death sentence.

I called my mom and sister before I talked with my husband. Their reactions were far from what I expected. They immediately began to speak faith, not fear, the complete opposite of what their first response would have been in times past. It blessed me how much their faith had grown and I knew I could count on their support.

As I shared with them my questions and concerns, what I heard was "All is well; faith not fear." To this day I have not thought any differently.

It was finally time to call my husband. He voiced what I had already heard from my sister and mom. "All is well; we will get through this." My heart ached for him and the fact that he would once again be thrown into the role of provider and caregiver, but something on the inside knew that if I had to go through this, then he is the one I wanted by my side!

Our daughter, Brittney, had told us just a few weeks earlier that she was pregnant with our first grandchild. So it took several days before I shared my diagnosis with her.

Since then, we now have two beautiful grandchildren: our little prince Noel who is three, and our princess Aria who just turned one.

While there are so many things that have taken place throughout all of this, I can truly say that God and His word, coupled with friends and family, and even complete strangers placed in my path, have been a source of strength and encouragement.

My journey after diagnosis began with a lumpectomy in December of 2012. Two weeks later, I was told that there were more cancer cells and I would need an additional surgery, so 28 days after the first surgery I was under the knife again having a mastectomy.

I finished chemotherapy that summer and then began several months of radiation.

It has taken a series of five surgeries to put "Patchwork Patti" – my affectionate name for myself – back together again.

My testimony is that, through all of this, I can still smile. My faith never wavered. I am so very thankful for the friends, family, coworkers and strangers I have met along the way.

So now it's my turn to pay it forward. Cancer treatment stripped away a lot of layers of the "me" I thought I needed to be.

Now with the new me, I work harder at trying to pay attention to life and those around me. My 2nd Act after my journey has allowed me to become a life coach for women who have areas in their lives where they are stuck, distracted, unfocused, unsure, and even unmotivated to change.

Through Healing Hearts Ministry, I offer my services

to those in my local church and those referred to me who do not attend. I've found that sickness and disease are not the only distractors that cause us to get off track and lose our identity and life purpose. We as women spend so much time caring for others, that we fail ourselves.

I have a friend who found herself in that rut for a while when she ran across a book called The Intentional Woman by an Arizona author. She introduced me to the book. Together we were so impressed by how it was impacting our own lives, we created a group that will come together for six weeks, helping women unpack their issues, find the power of their story and help them to live it out loud.

While I find it very rewarding to help others, I in no way profess to have it all together. What I do profess is that I refuse to stay down and I ALWAYS fight to get back up and find a 2nd Act.

So what did I do with that slip of mine that was hanging?

I took it off! I wave it now as my flag, my reminder that what I thought mattered doesn't. And what I was concerned that people would see is exactly what they NEED to see. I am a walking testament that no matter what comes your way, you can weather the storm!

CHAPTER 16

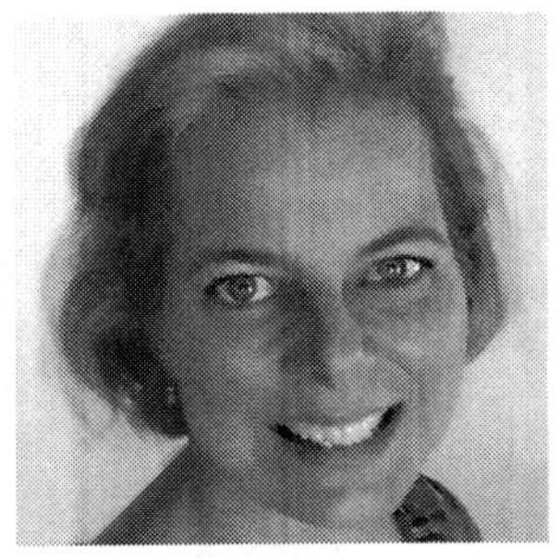

SARA THERESE MOORE

AML Cancer Survivor

Sara is a photographer, artist, writer, and now - cancer survivor. With the soul of a gypsy, she's backpacked through 29 countries on five continents; most recently traveling solo in a 17 foot travel trailer. She has chosen to share her leukemia journey as part of her travel blog, Sarandipity Travels, hoping her transparency in writing will help others cope with their own struggles. Learn more at www.sarandipitytravels.com

I'm very new to being a cancer survivor, but not new to surviving. You see, I watched my mother battle leukemia from the time I was 10 years old until I laid in bed with her as a teenager and watched her take her last breath.

In 2004, I found my son, shortly after his 15th birthday, dead on the couch due to suicide. This was followed by my sister's passing in 2010, and most recently, my husband's death in January of this year while I was in the midst of fighting my newly diagnosed cancer.

I can tell you this with a peaceful heart, because each loved one has had a profound impact on me. In their life and in their death, they have helped to shape who I am.

And I like who I am. Long ago I stopped asking "Why me?" I live by the motto, "It is what it is, but it will become what you make of it."

While talking with my daughter one day last fall, shortly after my diagnosis, she encouraged me to share my cancer journey with the world through my blog: Sarandipity Travels.

I took her advice and my hope has been that being transparent in my writing will help others cope with their own struggles. It is a part of my 2nd Act.

We all have a story to tell and being vulnerable enough to bare our souls so we can be fully embraced and understood, is one of the most beautiful experiences in life. Please allow me to share some of my blog entries with you.

Oct. 9th, 2015
Day 5 and still no diagnosis ....
I lay in the dark in my hospital room, silent tears rolling down my face. They follow the path of previous tears and I don't bother to wipe them away.

Yesterday was my hardest day. It started with a wave of dizziness, followed by pain in my chest, as I struggled to get my breath. A rush of doctors and nurses surrounded me, while my father and stepmom stood quietly to one side. A respiratory therapist tried to give me a mask but my hand shook and I couldn't find my face.

Later, I could hear my step-mom asking questions of the hospitalist quietly outside the cracked door.

"I'm sorry. She's very, very sick," was the only response I heard.

Now, in the quiet of the night, I cried… not for myself, but for my daughter and parents. I knew what it meant to lose a mother, and I knew what it meant to lose a child. It wasn't supposed to be like this.

The blue of the night was replaced by the warm light of dawn peeking through the crooked slats of my window. The flow of doctors and nurses would soon begin, each entering my room with masks and kind eyes that hinted at their hidden smiles.

Sprinkled between these visits were medications, blood draws, bone marrow biopsies, and the sound of my family's cheerful voices. They told stories to fill the silent hours and lighten the heaviness that crowded the corners of my thoughts.

The soft spoken oncologist entered my room and I could see it pained him to tell me he didn't have news on my biopsy yet. For the next half an hour, he answered all of the questions I asked; questions based in fear followed by answers I didn't hear.

Day 11 and two young doctors confirm my suspicion of leukemia. They smiled when they told me I had acute promyelocytic leukemia, and at first I thought their upbeat demeanor was a way of softening the bad news. But they seemed truly excited.

"You don't understand. This is a good thing! This is the most curable form of AML leukemia there is! It's very aggressive, but also very rare and very treatable." In that moment, I began to sob. These were tears of joy, and I said the most heartfelt prayer I've ever said. "Thank you, God!"

Dec. 25th, 2015
I spent Christmas morning getting chemo. My treatment plan calls for 110 chemo infusions and there were no breaks for holidays. I was given the beautiful gift of poison, wrapped in a clear plastic bag, hanging on a pole just for me; a gift bag of arsenic that I'm so

thankful to receive. It made me think about the irony of it all.

Society loves a triumphant, positive hero. It makes us feel good to see someone fight and win, and stay strong through it all.
It's much harder to see someone rage, and fall apart, and admit they're struggling. This scenario puts pressure on the cancer patient to bury their emotions for the benefit of others.

To state the obvious, "this isn't easy!" I'm human, and weak, and often get down in the muck and wallow at how horrible it is.

I get why people resent the word 'gift' and 'cancer' used in the same sentence. Yet after each mud bath of frustration and anger, I slog my way toward the positives. I reach my muddy hand out to receive the gifts because they help me to heal my torn bits.

So what are my gifts of cancer? I've been shown the beauty of the human spirit. Unselfish, compassionate human beings have appeared in abundance. If I ever questioned my worth in this world, I will never do so again. I know I'm loved.

I let the trivial fall away, cherish authentic relationships, live and speak my truth. I'm quick to hug, and slow to leave. I value kindness above all else.

We don't know when our time on this earth will end.

Cancer took the distant death deadline that I never thought about, and shoved it in my face for examination.

Remission has allowed me to distance myself from the inevitable once again, but keeps my mortality present enough to appreciate each day.

In a very real and powerful way, I know that today is a gift and in my 2nd Act, I recognize the perfection in all experiences.

Now, I travel the nation, a solo female in her tiny travel trailer, camera in one hand, pen and paper in another, experiencing life to it's fullest and sharing a piece of my soul with others, in the hopes that they, too, can create a 2nd Act after their life struggles.

The good news is that none of these lessons need come from experiencing cancer. In fact, much of this I already knew. But, leukemia has been the catalyst in reminding me: To Love. To feel. To travel. To take risks. To be gentle with myself. And ultimately, to connect on a deeper level.

Thank you, Cancer. Now, get lost!

CHAPTER 17

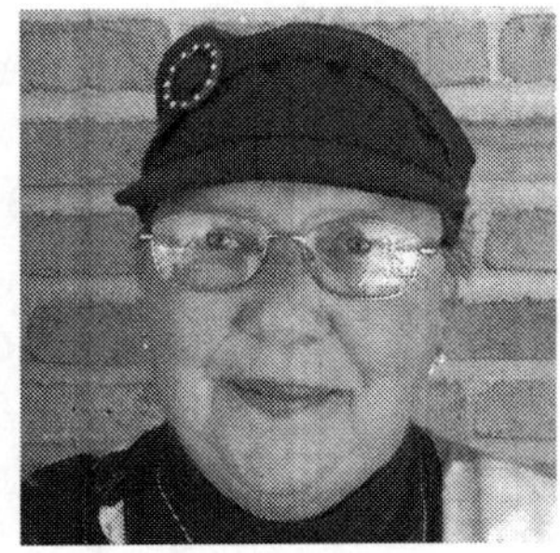

ISABELLE SUE BARBOUR

Breast and Ovarian Cancer Survivor

Isabelle's first book, *A Woman Under Construction*, offers readers a road map of her journey through diagnosis and treatment for breast cancer. Now in treatment for ovarian cancer, Isabelle thanks her family and especially her husband, Duane-Rafe, for all the years of help and support.

CHAPTER 17: ISABELLE SUE BARBOUR

The most shattering phone call I've ever received came in 2005. "I'm so sorry, Isabelle," said my doctor. "It's breast cancer. You will have to go to surgery." Thus started an odyssey that continues to this day.

The next step took my husband and me to a cancer center where, as far as I could tell, everyone was speaking in tongues. They seemed to think we should be in a hurry to understand what they were telling us.

There were unfamiliar medical terms, strange sounding tests, options for surgical procedures, clinical trials. On and on the new information went, mostly over our heads. The only thing we heard for sure was that I had a very aggressive type of cancer and didn't have the luxury of dithering around. It had to go.

Decisions had to be made on the spot. A lot of labs, x-rays and tests had to be done, all of which would culminate in some type of devastating surgery. And all in the next few days. I've spent more time dallying over the selection of a new car than on the choices I needed to make to ensure that I would have a future.

Frantic, I visited the cancer center's library in hopes of some guidance from other patients. Prowling the shelves, I looked for information that would help me decide which procedure would be best for me. But sadly, I found no patient stories of any kind.

"Okay," I thought to myself. "If I can't find a road map that works, why don't I create one for other patients coming after me?" And that's exactly what I did, never realizing that I was starting my 2nd Act in the process.

As I proceeded through experimental surgery and chemotherapy, I wrote about what I found along the way. I journaled about what having cancer can do TO you, and as time went by I realized some things about what having cancer can do FOR you.

For instance, I soon learned that cancer doesn't happen just to the patient. It happens to the whole family, to friends, co-workers, neighbors. Everyone feels the impact of a loved one getting cancer.

I wrote it all down, with no clue that I was giving birth to a book. I called it A Woman Under Construction. My original intention was to simply write something to be available to patients in that cancer center's particular library. But thanks to well-meaning friends, my little story found a publisher and wandered off on its own.

Soon I began receiving cards and emails from around the country. I read precious letters thanking me: for helping someone understand a loved one's illness; for helping someone find courage and hope; for unraveling the confusion of a new diagnosis.

Passed hand to hand, my book went where it was needed, with very little help from me. Too ill to participate in any sort of marketing, each letter lifted my own tortured heart and gave me a sense of wonder that my story had helped people navigate the minefields of a cancer diagnosis.

Perhaps the most poignant moment of my whole life occurred one day at a street fair, when a young lady bounced up and threw her arms around me. "I had to meet you," she said. "I saw your picture in that book, A Woman Under Construction." Startled, I agreed that I was indeed the lady in the picture.

"I knew it!" she said. "I want you to know that book saved my life. I couldn't face the thought of having cancer and had decided to go ahead and die. But the social worker brought me your book and asked me to read it before I decided.

"I did, and thought, 'Hey, if she can do it, so can I.' So I had the surgery and all the treatment." She went on, "I just wanted you to meet my husband and our baby, and to thank you for sharing your courage with others."

Turning, she walked away with her husband's arm around her, cure behind her, and her life back. Dumbfounded, I decided I had just heard the best book review there could ever be.

Around that time, I had found that I carry the BRCA gene, and suddenly I was fighting to survive metastatic ovarian cancer. My prognosis was very poor. Simultaneously, my beloved daughter was diagnosed with breast cancer.

Together we went to chemo loaded with craft projects to see us through those difficult times. We said, "If we are still alive by Christmas, at least we'll have the presents ready!" PAUSE I'm happy to say that my daughter lives, and just celebrated her five-year milestone. As for me, having ovarian cancer is like having a deadbeat relative. It keeps coming back, PAUSE with its grubby hand out, ready to take more than I have to give. I'm currently on my fifth recurrence. Maybe I'm really just a stubborn old broad, PAUSE but I like to think of myself as a survivor!

It's a hard row to hoe, that's true. Sometimes I lose track of which surgeries I had when, or how many kinds of chemotherapies I've taken. I often forget whether my hair is coming or going PAUSE as I progress through treatment after treatment.

Sometimes I get so tired I would cheerfully lie down on the floor in Walmart if my pride would let me.

Even my own brother said to me, "Boy you sure are taking a long time to die!" PAUSE You gotta love brothers – and I love mine!

But I live, and I love my life every time I see another Christmas or another birthday. A gorgeous morning, or a new baby in the family. Each event is a win; each day is another miracle.

And when I'm worn out in strength or spirit, I think of those cards and letters from places like Tampa and

Bowling Green and Milwaukee, and especially that sweet young lady in Little Rock.

My gift to other cancer patients came right back home to uplift and encourage me to write another book. God willing, my 2nd act will bring comfort and hope to even more people.

CHAPTER 18

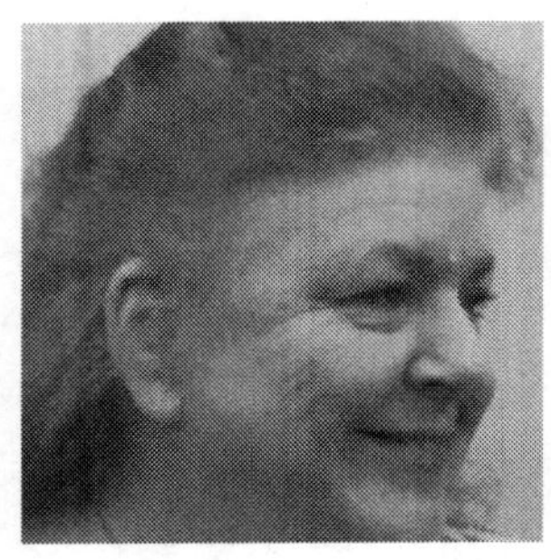

KAREN CONWAY

Ovarian Cancer Survivor

Karen was diagnosed three times with ovarian cancer – 11, 10 and nine years ago. She is a member of the Tucson chapter of the National Ovarian Cancer Coalition, helping to bring awareness to this silent killer: "It whispers, so listen." She also attends two other support groups helping others on their cancer journeys.

CHAPTER 18: KAREN CONWAY

Lying in bed in a corner suite, like some kind of a princess. Ha – I didn't even have medical insurance! I kept repeating it over and over. I have cancer ... I have ovarian cancer. OH MY GOD! I'm gonna die! God please don't let me die; I'll do anything you ask!

Like a whirlwind, a haboob, really, there was surgery, chemo, lab tests, CAT scans, MRI's, and new doctors' appointments. Plus, I didn't have a working cell. I couldn't call any of my family since most lived out of town, but they eventually found me.

During treatment, I found a cancer support group.

Two groups, actually, one for gynecological cancers specifically and the other for all women's cancers. What a relief to find other women with similar diagnoses and stories like mine. I don't know what I would have done without them. I've made lifelong friendships from them! They were a blessing beyond compare

My employment situation, on the other hand, was far less than a blessing. Despite my pleas, I lost my temp job because I could not return to work full time immediately after major surgery. Wait, what? That can't be right. I have cancer. I just had major cancer surgery! Can they do that? Apparently they can and did.

Despite my cancer fallout, I refound my passion – and what would become my 2nd Act – music! I had been involved in choral groups in North Caroline before I moved to Tucson.

First, I joined a women's choral group. Despite chemo and being immune-suppressed, I made rehearsals and even performed in concert with them, bald head and all! (Although I think I wore a scarf.)

Within a year I found a wonderful church choir, led by a doctor of music. Good, I thought, he'll demand it from us, which is what I had previously been used to. But best of all, they were planning a trip to New York City in May of 2007.

Remember the old joke, "How do you get to Carnegie Hall? PRACTICE! PRACTICE! PRACTICE!"

To sing at Carnegie Hall would be a dream come true, a bigger dream than I ever expected in my 2nd Act. Chemo was temporarily stopped and despite being somewhat debilitated from my treatment, I made the trip.

It was so exciting to sing Vivaldi's "Gloria" in that gorgeous hall, where so many famed vocalists and instrumentalists had performed before us. I sat there taking it all in ... ahh ... the ambience of Carnegie Hall. Wow!

Recurrence happened one year after my chemo ended and I followed the same gold standard for treatment again. I lost my hair again, but I developed the attitude of, "Hey you did this once, you can do it again!" And lucky me, as a result of the ovarian cancer I developed Deep Vein Thromboses, which closed up some of the veins in my lower legs. It's a chronic disability, and nothing can be done to improve that. Hence my companion the cane.

Six months after my second diagnosis, I got my third hit: metastases to the brain. I opted for radiation and got zapped with all they had in just one session.

Repeated MRIs, CT and PET scans found my microscopic brain growth unchanged, yet kinda fuzzy. Had it grown? Had necrosis – tissue death – set in? Was it a reaction to the radiation?

More tests and finally a determination: it was tissue death from the radiation. And fortunately I had plenty of other brain tissue to make up for the dead stuff.

Finally some good news! The director of the church choir I sang with founded the Arizona Choral Society. Ahhh … choral masterworks. I was in heaven and I hadn't even died yet.

I eventually came to the conclusion that my cancer was a gift. It took me several years to admit that, and especially to say it out loud.

Not only have I made many incredible friendships, but I rediscovered my passion for music. Both have kept me alive all these many years later.

I fully understand that one can never return to what life was exactly like before cancer, but that's not so bad. We call it the "new normal," And "new normal" can apply to anyone in any situation. What have you always wanted to try but were afraid to tackle? What passion do you have that you want to rediscover, like I did with my music?

I'm here to tell you the sky's the limit – go for it!

PHOENIX

Spring in the desert is filled with magical sights and sounds. So it is with survivorship, as each of these Valley of the Sun women survivors found magic and miracles in the wake of the world's most dreaded disease. Their stories are testaments to a phrase often repeated by survivors: "Cancer was a gift."

Sunday, March 12, 2017, 2:00 p.m.
Mesa Arts Center, Mesa, AZ

This performance was made possible by the generosity of Cancer Treatment Centers of America, Scottsdale Medical Imaging, Ltd., Ironwood Cancer Research Center, Mosharrafa Plastic Surgery, and Kendra Scott Jewelry.

Love to Dave Pratt, Emcee, Founder of Star Worldwide Networks

CHAPTER 19

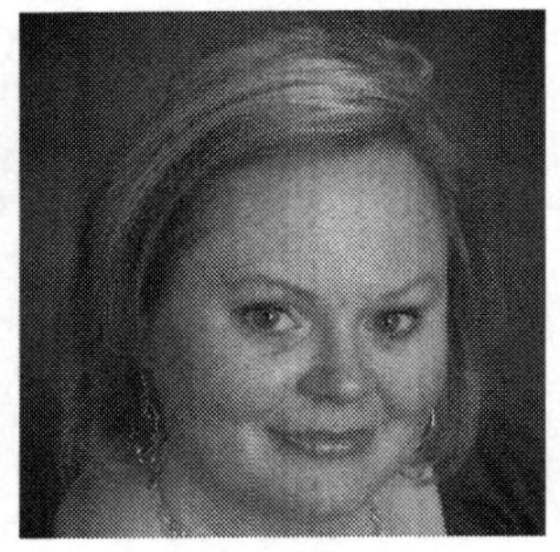

KARI GROVES

Thyroid Cancer Survivor

Kari is a native Arizonan, a wife, and the mother of two beautiful daughters. She serves as Program Man-ager for Singleton Moms, a local nonprofit organization dedicated to serving the needs of single parents battling cancer and their minor children. She embraces the organization's motto, "Meeting the needs of today and providing hope for tomorrow." Learn more at www.singletonmoms.org.

Thank you so much
for all your done for
a 2nd Act!

Kari Groves...

Papillary Thyroid Cancer – the "best cancer," they said, if you have to have cancer.

Picture this. It was 2004. I was 28 years old, a newly married wife and the mother of a two-year-old. On a Wednesday morning, I went into my doctor's office with a sore throat, where upon they found a lump the size of a golf ball. A biopsy followed on Friday, and I was immediately scheduled for the removal of my entire thyroid the following Monday. This would remove "the best cancer to have."

The surgery was effective, with only a couple of complications.

A month later, I received the I-131 radioactive iodine treatment which was prescribed to treat all the remaining nodules. This would completely eradicate "the best cancer to have."

Only it didn't. Over the course of the next four years, "the best cancer to have" came back, forcing me to endure three more excruciatingly difficult rounds of radiation treatment. Each one isolated me in a plastic lined hospital room resembling a giant Ziplock bag, for an entire week. I was kept from my daughter and any contact with my husband or family.

And then, after my third treatment, and against my doctor's orders, we got pregnant. We are now the proud parents of two amazingly beautiful daughters.

Apparently, I'll never be rid of "the best cancer to have." Since 2008, I have received regular six-month scans and oncology visits to watch the metastasis continue to grow. It happens at such a slow rate that removal isn't an option. And I've reached my lifetime limit of treatment of radioactive iodine treatments. Any more and I would likely contract leukemia.

So I wait, and plan for my family's future. But my cancer journey has allowed me to create an incredible 2nd Act!

In 2010, at the gentle and loving suggestion of my husband, I enrolled to get my Master's Degree in Nonprofit Management and Leadership. This in turn has allowed me to pursue greater and increasingly more meaningful and impactful work.

While living in Seattle, I became a Parents As Teachers Home Visitor with Friends of Youth. I mentored young, first time parents and their children to foster loving and educational relationships.

At the same time, I was also the Director of Children's Education at Bellevue First Congregational Church, designing and facilitating weekly teacher trainings, staff development and the loving education of our community's most vulnerable youth.

Life's journey is interesting, isn't it? Those work experiences, and having "the best cancer to have," prepared me for what has unfolded the last two years.

In early 2015, without warning, our oldest daughter was struck over night with a debilitating and mysterious illness. It left our beautiful 13-year-old bed-ridden and in the fight for her life.

It started with persistent and unrelenting migraine-type headaches that continue to this day. She was diagnosed with Lyme's disease, which many physicians deem improbable and "fake."

Simultaneously she contracted fibromyalgia. Almost overnight, she lost the use of her limbs.

My husband and I, along with our entire family, each found our own methods of coping with her illness. But it was my first-hand cancer journey that guided me to process my daughter's situation in a unique and profound way.

Her illness brought our family closer than I ever thought possible. I'm happy to report she has improved immensely and is now functioning at almost 100%. And I have found yet another direction for my 2nd Act!

Incorporating my love for children and their families, along with "the best cancer to have," I am now the Program Manager for a local nonprofit organization called Singleton Moms. I lead a team of dedicated employees and volunteers, as we meet the families' needs of today and provide hope for their tomorrow.

Eleven years ago, our founder, Jody Farley, helped a high school friend named Michelle Singleton. Michelle was a single mom of four children when diagnosed with Stage IV breast cancer at a very young age.

After Michelle died, Jody recognized there had to be more parents in the Valley with Michelle's needs. Singleton Moms started on Jody's kitchen counter and now assists single parents battling cancer, and their minor children, throughout Maricopa County.

In my role, and using my personal experiences, I have had the incredible honor of honing programs that are uniquely structured for these families at their darkest time.

Our work is varied and vast. We partner with a local commercial kitchen called Dream Dinners to create 190 nutritious, gourmet and healthy meals for our families every month. Each meal is prepared by our volunteers.

And in coordination with Jody, I am spearheading a program for pediatric cancer patients and their families. This will include a support network for this unique population, all the while maintaining our core programs.

I am passionate about spreading our mission and our vision with community members, volunteers, donors and parents alike. Part of my 2nd Act is to make sure that we can gather and support as many families as possible. And being a part of this cast has magnified that potential. We even have a former Singleton Mom recipient in this cast!

Could I do this work simply with my degree? Probably. But would I be as effective and whole-heartedly compassionate without my own cancer journey? Doubtful.

Clearly "the best cancer to have" really has been!

CHAPTER 20

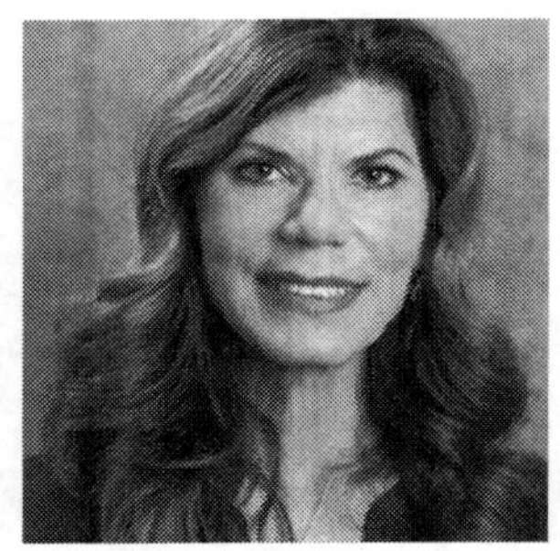

NANCY LITTERMAN HOWE

Squamous Cell Cancer Survivor

Nancy was a daily exerciser who ate her fruits and vegetables. But in 1997, she was diagnosed with cancer anyway. She experienced first-hand the benefits of physical activity during treatment and beyond. That was her "Aha!" moment. She left her corporate career, returned to school, and founded www.StrongCancerRecovery.org.

Hello! I am definitely the vaudeville portion of today's program. Let me explain how I came to be on the stage today.

In 2013 I created my 2nd Act when I founded my non-profit, Strong Cancer Recovery. I have one focus: advocate for exercise to become part of the Standard of Care for oncology treatment.

I believed then, and I believe even more strongly now, that change will come when cancer patients loudly request exercise programs from their oncologists, and oncologists press their administrators for in-house exercise facilities for their patients.

Part of my work is to speak at cancer-related events, where I describe my own cancer diagnosis and treatment, and the research-proven benefits of exercise for people living with a diagnosis of cancer. I distribute resistance bands and teach exercises too.

In 2015, I spoke at a dozen events, reaching nearly 800 survivors and oncologists. But I wanted to reach more. A year ago, I learned of an opportunity for me to reach nearly 900 seniors in a single night. All I needed to do was enter the Ms. Senior Arizona pageant, and turn my 20-minute advocacy talk into a two-and-a-half-minute talent.

Which I did.

So while the other 20 contestants were dressed in elegant gowns and singing, or wearing top hats and tails as they tap-danced, I took the stage, dressed like this, and explained the benefits of exercise for cancer survivorship to the full auditorium of 925!

Although my talent was highly unconventional, the judges clearly got it. Like me, they saw the value in my message being delivered to as many seniors as possible. I placed third overall, and during that one week, I spoke to more than 1100 seniors in Phoenix's West Valley.

I know that the groundswell demand from patients for structured exercise programs will continue to grow. It is my hope that, as a group, oncologists will make time during clinical visits to emphasize to their patients the importance of physical activity.

Research suggests that patients are twice as likely to start exercising if their oncologist recommends it. We're not re-creating the wheel here. We just need to get it rolling!

These days, when I speak, I remind oncologists that it doesn't take much time or a deep knowledge of exercise physiology to make this recommendation.

In fact, my two-and-a-half minute talent at the Ms. Senior Arizona Contest is exactly what I want oncologists to promote.

My passion is teaching magic. Let me tell you why.

In 1997 I was 42, a daily exerciser, and I ate my fruits and vegetables. I got cancer anyway.

It was aggressive – a rapidly growing, golf-ball-sized tumor in my throat. Treatment was aggressive too, and exhausting, with gruesome side effects.

My surgery removed the roof of my mouth, creating a cavernous echo chamber for my voice.

The radiation dried up my salivary glands. Let me assure you that saliva is a very under-rated body fluid. For the first three years following treatment, my meal plans included protein shakes, oatmeal, and ice-cream. Not all bad!

But back then, they couldn't target radiation like they can now, so my head and neck radiation was also carotid artery and heart radiation, for which I see a cardiac specialist, despite my active lifestyle.

I could also tell you about the disastrous effects on my teeth – again no saliva – which cost about the same as a Mercedes convertible, and not nearly as much fun.

But when I came through far better than expected, my oncologist guessed it was because I was so fit when we started treatment.

My diagnosis, and strong recovery, gave me a mission.

At 51, I earned my master's degree in exercise at Arizona State University. And today, 11 years later, I work with the oncology team at Mayo Clinic.

I teach cancer patients that exercise reduces their risk of relapse, lessens the long-term side effects of treatment, and combats depression.

Most of my patients are 50 and older. Most already feel terrible about themselves for not exercising enough. That's when I teach them the magic of exercise.

You see, the benefits of exercise are cumulative. Even if we can only exercise for two minutes before we have to stop and rest. I point out that two minutes every hour in an eight hour day is 16 minutes of exercise. And 16 minutes is more than half of the 30 minutes recommended by the Surgeon General.

That's success! That feels like magic!

So what do we do for two minutes that makes such a difference?

We sit down, and we stand up. We sit down, we stand up, we sit down, we stand UP.

And how much do we do? More than the day before. And really, that's all that's needed to trigger the benefits of exercise for anybody.

So I ask you, "Isn't that a kind of magic?"

But there's more to my 2nd Act. Last month, I was hired by Arizona State University to research the very subject I've been so passionate about.

As a Research Specialist Senior, I'll be able to truly contribute to the science I've long known improves and saves lives.

Now that's magic!

CHAPTER 21

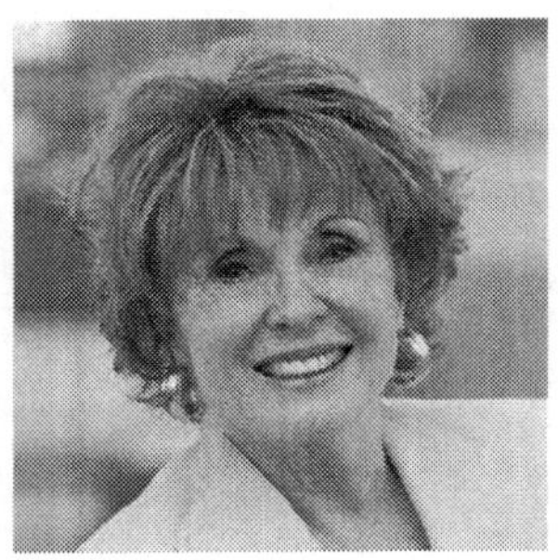

SUE ELLEN ALLEN

Breast Cancer Survivor

Sue Ellen Allen is an activist, speaker and author whose remarkable journey through cancer introduced her to a life's purpose that took her to the White House. She is the founder of www.ReinventingReentry.org and the author of *The Slumber Party From Hell*, a memoir of turning tragedy to triumph.

Make a difference!

Sue Ellen

Valentine's Day, 2002, I was diagnosed with stage 3B breast cancer. My prognosis was less than five years. My treatment would be chemotherapy, followed by surgery.

Then suddenly, that July, humiliated and disgraced, I entered the Maricopa County jail to await sentencing for securities fraud.

I went to my mastectomy shackled, handcuffed and belly chained. No friends or family present. No one touched me but the surgeons with their knives, the nurses with their needles and the guards with their handcuffs.

I'd lost 28 lymph nodes along with my breast and the surgeon issued an order to the jail for a pillow to cushion and protect my arm from lymphedema.
Order denied. No pillows were allowed in the jail.

When I got back from the hospital, women packed into my cell to see how I was. Breaking a huge rule, they hugged me, the first hugs I'd received. Aren't hugs wonderful?

These tough women were so upset about the pillow rule, they left my cell grumbling. A few hours later they were back with an order of their own. "Close your eyes, Sue Ellen, and hold out your hands."

When I did, I felt the softest thing: it was the most

beautiful pillow I have ever seen, light blue, tufted and fringed, and it did not come in a Tiffany bag.

Where on earth? Then I realized it was made of the Kotex pads furnished by the jail! These tough women had contributed their precious supplies and woven them together into a tufted square.

They used the small golf pencil that's allowed for a writing tool to punch holes in the ends of the pads. They shredded thin strips from another pad to use as thread to sew it all around. Finally, they fringed it to give it that designer look.

At the darkest time in my life, drug addicts, prostitutes, and murderers looked after me, and I will NEVER forget them.

March 18, 2009, I was finally free. I started working in the criminal justice system because I found my purpose and my 2nd Act in prison. In eight years I've worked to bring education inside the women's prison. And I've worked to bring education outside to the general public, by drawing attention to the horror of our prison system, especially if you're sick.

I watched my cell mate die of leukemia because the prison kept denying her a simple blood test.

She was so sick and when they finally took her to the hospital, her red blood count was 300,000 and her white blood count was ZERO.

I'd never seen a body shut down. The pain was excruciating. Gina was only 25. Her three year sentence became a death sentence.

After her death, I asked if we could have a cancer walk in October. I didn't know it had NEVER been done before. The prison staff looked at me like I had three heads, but they finally agreed.

We decorated the yard with pink construction paper – the place looked like a Pepto Bismol explosion! We walked around and around the track, and raised $10,000 from inmates and staff for the American Cancer Society. That was in 2003 and that walk is still going on in Arizona prisons, raising money for cancer.

If you had told me before I went to prison what I'd see and experience, I would have said, "Not in our country. We don't treat people that way." I was wrong. We do, and being sick is especially terrifying.

So my 2nd Act is to educate the public about this draconian $80 billion business. America is the incarceration nation, incarcerating more people per capita than Russia or China.

In prison, I encountered a lot of single mothers, there because of addiction. Their children were being raised by others. In America, 1 in 28 children now has a parent in prison. In America, every 26 seconds, a child drops out of school. In America, one in three people has a criminal record. How is that acceptable in America?

January 3, 2016, seven years after I was freed. I was waiting for Downton Abby to start. My phone rang. ID unknown. I don't answer ID unknown. Rang again. Ignored it. Rang AGAIN. This time voice mail. OK, I'll listen.

"Ms. Allen, this is XYZ at the White House calling. Would you please call me back as soon as possible?"

Oh sure, the White House calling ME. I don't think so. Did you know you can Google the White House? Nice operators 24/7. So I called just to verify it wasn't a hoax. I gave them the name left on my voice mail. "Yes ma'm, that's one of our staffers." OK, I thought. I guess I'd better call back.

The call was an invitation to be one of 23 Americans to sit in the First Lady's box at President Obama's final State of the Union address. I was to represent criminal justice reform. I was very cool.

"You know I'm an ex-felon?" "Yes, ma'am, we know all about you."

A week later I was on a whirlwind trip to Washington, D.C., where I was interviewed by NBC in front of the White House and the BBC on the radio. I met with the Attorney General Loretta Lynch. Me, a former inmate.

I attended a gorgeous reception at the White House. It seemed more like a movie than real life.

I met Mrs. Obama and Dr. Biden, then rode in a motorcade to the capitol, sirens blazing.

Looking down from the First Lady's box in the historic chamber of the House of Representatives, I could see all of our Congressional leaders, the Supreme Court Justices, the Cabinet and Joint Chiefs of Staff. Just like on TV.

Then in a flash it was over. Our security detail came to escort us, I thought, to the motorcade back to the White House. But instead, they took us into a long hallway where we waited and waited.

Finally, I asked why. "Don't you know, Sue Ellen?" came the response from another person who'd been in the box with me. "We're going to meet the President and have our picture taken!"

Oh my goodness. My first thought was pure vanity: my lipstick is in my purse, in the limousine in the motorcade!

We inched up to the door and then it was my turn. There stood the President.

He beamed and gave me a huge hug and I thanked him for visiting a prison last summer. We had a brief chat then he turned me just right to make sure the picture was perfect. And it was.

In June of last year, I was invited back to speak on a panel on criminal justice at a White House sponsored summit, "The United State of Women."

In November, I went back one more time to speak to a group of leaders in justice reform. Led by the Attorney General and Presidential Advisor Valerie Jarrett, their message inspired us to continue our work and never give up on our purpose and our vision.

Do you make New Year's resolutions or set goals. I don't, but if I did, never EVER would I have set a goal that one day I would be in the First Lady's box at the State of the Union in our nation's Capitol. That's like saying, I'm going to win an Oscar without ever being in a movie!

It's what I call God's magic. It's the reason we can never give up. Life can change in an instant to terrify you, like when you hear the words, "You've got cancer." It can also change instantly to thrill you. Like when the White House calls and the result gives your 2nd Act the kind of power and attention it deserves. It's God's magic.

I ask you ALL to remember God's magic and God's message that after cancer and often because of cancer, there is life and purpose and passion.

ALL of these women here are examples that cancer

can give us the power to grow stronger so we can Show Up, Speak Up and Do Stuff in our 2nd Act!

CHAPTER 22

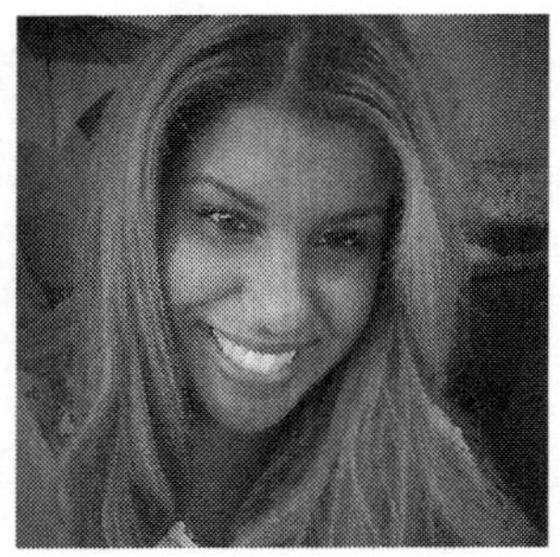

NADIA J. SAMUEL

Hodgkin's Lymphoma
Cancer Survivor

Nadia is certified in Cancer Peer Support through Arizona Cancer Survivors Circle of Strength, a community of cancer survivors and advocates who provide support to those touched by cancer. She is also an advocate for stress elimination through balance and meditation. As an entrepreneur, she has developed Stress Nano, which offers solutions anyone can achieve.

Learn more at www.StressNano.com.

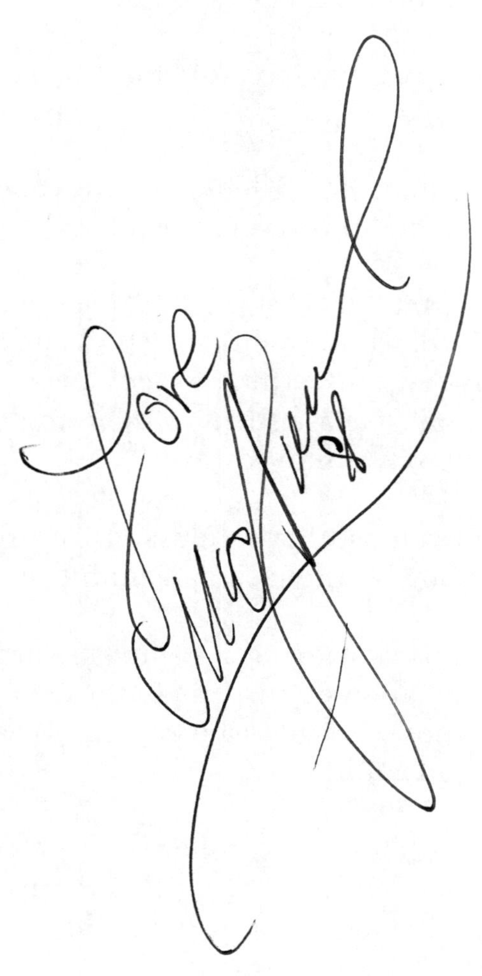

We all have a story, and it can be told in many ways -- through social media ... via frames lining the walls of our childhood bedrooms ... in the faces and expressions of the ones you count on as your support team or confidants ... or in a medical report.

Today I will try to capture my story for you, if only just for a few moments.

My 2nd Act began in 2007, when I became cancer free. This year marks my 10 year anniversary!

Within my 2nd Act, I feel I was gifted a new chance to discover my path, truly identifying who I am, helping to redefine my story, discerning which dreams belong solely to me, and to chase them to their end or until they weave themselves into reality.

And I realized you can have thousands of dreams! I do – and each one is unique and beautiful.

My cancer diagnosis came as a complete surprise. I mean, it's almost always a surprise to those of us who have been diagnosed. I had just turned 21. Woo - hoo! I was officially an adult.

On a quick visit home from college – for Mom's express laundry service and such – I found my mother in the kitchen. She looked at me and said, "Wow, you look horrible!"

Thanks, Mom.

"No really you should see a doctor," she said. The "I've-been-busy-and-I-have-a-lot-of-pressure-at-school" responses didn't quell her pushing. So I went the next day and came home with a smug smile.

"I just need to eat breakfast and take more vitamins." "Go see another doctor," my mother said.

Within 20 minutes into the exam with my new doctor – the one I chose out of the insurance book, with the most abbreviations next to her name, to keep my mom quiet – she said, "You have cancer. Cancel classes and let's get you to an oncologist right away."

Confirmed by five different oncologists, I had had Hodgkin's Lymphoma for two years already. I was at stage II, and tumors had begun to expand in two separate systems in my body.

Choosing a treatment plan and the right oncologist took much longer than diagnosis. The difficulty was due to the fact that I was a bit of a puzzle. Half of the doctors specialized in treating much older patients and the other half specialized in pediatrics.

Treatment protocols for each group varied considerably. Sitting in each waiting room, I felt out of place. I either stared at toys on the floor, or retirement ads while the doctors contemplated factors they usually didn't, like fertility or college classes. In the end, they tossed me into the pediatric group. There went my official adult pass!

There were some bumps during chemo. And with no support group for my age group, I was thankful and fortunate to have chosen an oncology team that truly understood my frustration at this juncture. They gave me a voice during treatment, and a special place of my own in their office.

After the flurry of treatment I navigated my new path in my 2nd Act, two main dreams became clearer and clearer as I grew into my new skin. Both had the same mission: to always reach out to those who need, to give them a hand as they make their way through their own stories.

The first dream, was to become a volunteer and peer support advocate for cancer patients and survivors.

As a volunteer, I hoped to contribute my stories, my mistakes, my tips and above all, hope.

And though I wished to help as many as possible, my passion was to gain as much experience as I could as a Peer Advocate. I wanted to help those who found themselves wedged in the generational gap, between pediatrics and a much older generation.

It is hard to believe that 10 years later, though treatment and access to information are dramatically enhanced, support for the young adult group – from a perspective they can relate to – has not improved much.

I was so ecstatic to find Arizona Cancer Survivors Circle of Strength, a volunteer community of cancer survivors, caregivers, friends and families who provide hope, strength, and support to those who have been touched by cancer.

This group has welcomed me with open arms, allowing me to explore this pursuit and I am truly grateful. They have given me the opportunity to obtain my Peer Support Certification as I embarked on my 2nd Act.

I support them by volunteering at events, runs and walks put on by partner organizations in our community. I am also excited to assist Circle of Strength with social media outreach and interaction within our community. I have joined their fundraising committee for 2017 and am writing exclusive pieces for their blog.

The board at Circle of Strength has been extremely supportive in my personal passion.

And with their guidance, I will pursue this dream until everyone in the young adult age group, whether patient or survivor, can say they have a fount of support that focuses on their needs.

My other 2nd Act mission focuses on a serious chronic illness that plagues millions of Americans every day, one for which it's hard to find help: chronic stress.

Yes, it is a lofty goal, but I believe with the right

support, we can all achieve a healthy state of balance, where our physical, mental, and emotional health are not plagued by daily recurrent, constant stress.

This dream has stemmed from my cancer experience.

Through cancer survivorship, I have witnessed the power of a support team, those who will go the extra mile to research alternative medicine, statistics on current treatments, and any clinical trials necessary to eliminate the disease so the patient can resume the life they were meant to have.

I believe that we should apply the same gusto and diligence toward eliminating stress. It can wreak havoc on our bodies, and in addition to mental health and emotional stability, it has even been linked to cancer.

From this passion, I created Stress Nano. I have assembled an expert team to develop a website and an app which will become a custom support team.

We are assembling every useful stress elimination method. They are intended to be a continuous solution, not simply a temporary state. We call this "stress release," instead of stress relief. When we feel relief, we're getting a temporary reprieve, but eventually the main source of the problem will rear its head. And then we seek temporary relief again and the cycle continues.

Our custom algorithm helps each user define the best

course of action in stress release suited to their profile.

Through a series of questions developed by specialists in psychology, yoga, massage therapy, education, meditation, nutrition, breath-work and mindfulness, users are able to get to the root of their stress. They can bypass solutions that may not be the most effective for them, and begin the release process immediately.

Users can also enhance their profiles and suggested solutions by entering or seamlessly integrating data from wireless devices such as heart rate monitors, fitness devices and even playlists!

This beloved project of mine will launch later this year. It combines so many things I love and find important: self-care, meditation, mindfulness, and other modalities. And it is an incredibly important agent in the fight against cancer.

So this is my 2nd Act. I will continuously strive to help as many as I can from as many perspectives that are available to me. I will dream for as long as I have this gift.

And my story will continue to be written.

CHAPTER 23

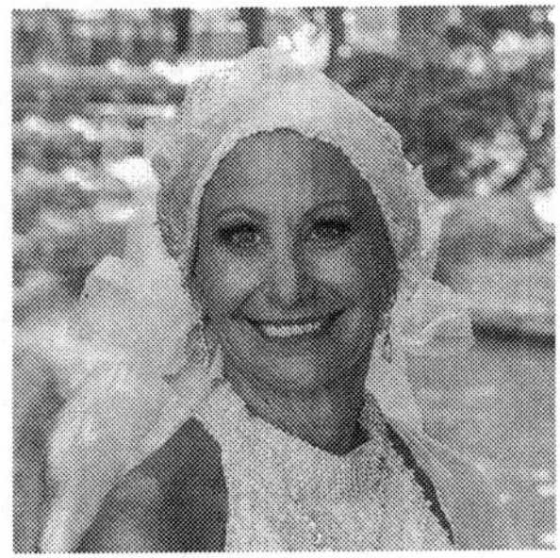

REBA MASON

Breast Cancer Survivor

This Texas girl lives in Surprise, AZ, and is the Founder and CEO of Reba's Vision. The organization provides free 3D digital mammograms to Phoenix area women, as well as wigs, prosthetics and bras free of charge to any woman in need while they are going through their cancer battle. Learn more at www.RebasVision.com.

CHAPTER 23: REBA MASON

My life has been filled with ups and downs, from being a Dallas Cowboys Cheerleader for four seasons, to battling an eating disorder that nearly took my life in 2000 and successfully overcoming it.

For my 40th birthday, my mom had given me the unique present of being tested to see if I carried the BRCA gene mutation. My grandmother, my mom, her twin sister, two cousins, and two other relatives had been diagnosed with either breast or ovarian cancer. Not surprisingly, I, too, carry the BRCA ER positive 2 gene mutation.

And then, on October 1, 2011, for better or worse, my first act ended for good. I had gone in for my six month mammogram. The doctor called and told me I needed to come in right away. I knew I had breast cancer, and indeed it was. They first thought it would be stage one. But in surgery, they discovered it was far more advanced. I had stage 3c invasive ductal carcinoma and awoke with a double mastectomy.

I knew this would forever change my life. My treatment was tough – 16 weeks of chemo, followed by 32 rounds of radiation. When that didn't work, the process was repeated. And then it was repeated again, for a total of 48 weeks of chemo and 96 rounds of radiation. Whew!

My chemo port became infected and was replaced three times, more cancer was discovered and I underwent surgery after surgery. But I knew I had to fight like a girl! And that became my motto.

At the same time, my mom, Marla Sue Mason, was battling stage 4 metastatic breast cancer. She had been fighting for 18 years and it came back four times, but she never gave up.

She volunteered at the center where she was receiving treatment and would tell everyone, "I don't have a terminal illness. I have a chronic illness that can be managed with treatment and faith." She fought like a girl, too, until she lost her battle on February 24, 2014.

Seven months later, in September of 2014, my life would begin its 2nd Act.

My amazing doctors informed me that my cancer had metastasized to my bones. My life expectancy was two to four years, maybe. Yes, I had my "why me" pity party that night. But at 2:00 a.m., I woke up, realizing I had had two visions.

Three weeks earlier, I had heard about a new type of mammogram, 3D digital tomography. It was reducing call-backs by 40%, and catching breast cancer up to 18 months earlier than a normal 2D mammogram.

I also learned that, without insurance, it cost a woman $111 to have this latest, more effective mammogram. I stared writing down cost times this, times that, and Reba's Vision was born!

If I could raise $3,000, I could maybe save 25 women from what I and so many others have gone through.

I also wanted to help women currently in treatment feel beautiful. And this was the second vision. I began providing them with a Basket of Hope. These baskets come from their surrounding community, and are filled with books, hats, makeup, jewelry, and anything else that gives them hope.

I had been given such items while I was undergoing my treatment. Little did I imagine that two years later, we would have raised nearly $100,000!

At the time, I was the marketing director at a Texas Roadhouse Restaurant, and the managing partner allowed me to turn the restaurant pink for the month of October. Over 100 women have used the Pink Roadhouse Mammo Fund.

In addition, Reba's Vision has provided more than 75 Hope Baskets.

My 2nd Act continues to grow as we now provide free wigs, bras, prosthetics, hats, scarves, anything a woman needs while in treatment for any form of cancer. It's all at no cost to them, through the generous donations from women who have been there and survived.

My 2nd Act is still going strong with the amazing support of my husband, who I met while battling cancer and married 11 months ago, and includes my family and countless friends, especially Gina Sheets.

I'm ready to begin my 3rd Act now. I will not let a little thing called cancer beat me. Because I know how to fight like a girl!

CHAPTER 24

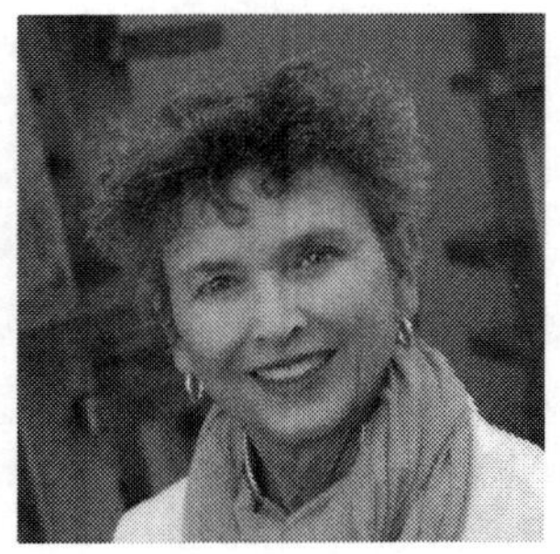

JAN COGGINS

Ovarian Cancer Survivor

Jan is a survivor, educator, spiritual leader, and the author of *Ovarian Cancer? You Can Not Be Serious!* A retired social worker who passionately advocates for ovarian cancer awareness, Jan's own cancer jour-ney keeps her motivated to find funds and resources for women with ovarian cancer through her organization the Teal It Up Foundation. Learn more at www.TealItUp.org.

CHAPTER 24: JAN COGGINS

Don't tell God the size of the mountain, tell the mountain the size of God.

Eight months after chemo for stage 3C ovarian cancer, and in celebration of my 60th birthday, I hiked 100 miles in the Swiss Alps. My gynecological oncologist said that I might be a little crazy when I told him I was hiking. But I did it anyway.

With neuropathy, it wasn't pretty. But along with my team of supporters, we made it. After that success, I got serious about survivorship.

Looking back over some of the cliffs I crossed in the Alps, I probably should have given some thought to survivorship then. But my mindset was that I had beaten cancer, and the mountains were next.

I am a seven-year survivor and thriver of ovarian cancer. And I consider that a feat greater than the mountain climbing. I live grate-FULL every day for life after such a diagnosis. Especially since I have lost more friends to this disease than I can bear to share.

It's been though faith, will, strength and the desire to help another person face this kind of adversity that I have found my way.

So many people had helped me during my journey that I wanted to give back. Every time I saw someone I thought might be in treatment, I'd approach them.

And before you knew it, we had a wonderful connection.

I felt like I could be a lightning rod to change the way they looked at their cancer. I told them to have the attitude of "Yes, I have cancer, but it doesn't have me;" "I am full of life, not cancer;" "See me, not it." I rocked the attitude that I would beat cancer and I want every other cancer patient to do the same.

My recurrence in 2012 hit hard, because I was so into rocking my survivorship. It took every fiber of my soul to stay on track and not go down the proverbial black hole.

Before my recurrence, I had begun writing a book entitled "Ovarian Cancer: You Can Not Be Serious!" It was launched in the spring of 2013, while I was still in chemo. And to my amazement, the book has been successful. I continue to receive emails from women across the country.

But I wanted to do more. So I formed the Teal It Up Foundation. Now, starting a foundation is sort of like hiking the Alps – crazy! But we have reached thousands, and given over $100,000 toward research for a cure to ovarian cancer.

Losing board members to the disease has been hugely impactful on me and the other board members. So in the past year, we decided to keep our funds local to help women within Arizona. We offer comfort bags to newly diagnosed and recurring gynecological cancer patients.

But one of the most rewarding programs we've started is our pet therapy program. Please meet Bozeman.

He was certified at the age of one to visit chemo rooms and hospitals by referral. Bozeman moves from patient to patient, hanging out with them and always near enough for them to love on him. The patients are held captive by their chemo lines. But he brings them such joy that his visits are highly requested.

If I could bottle the joy he brings to me and others, well … suffice it to say, I'd be in the Caribbean right now!

He's as much a part of my continued healing and well being as he is to those he meets during his day job.

But there's something else I'm as passionate about as Bozeman – genetic testing. There was no cancer in my family and in 2012, when I was BRCA tested, I was negative for the mutation. But new gene mutations were discovered and I was retested in 2015.

This time, I was positive for the PALB 2 mutation, which puts me at higher risk for pancreatic, breast and ovarian cancers. And here's the kicker. Both my sisters were tested and they're both positive as well.

Why am I telling you this? Genetic research and testing can mean the difference between life and death for many. So the Teal It Up Foundation funds anyone unable to pay for testing, if it's been deemed medically indicated. Some of the women we've helped have been found positive. I know those test results made a difference in their treatment options.

Now I'm not a public speaker. I grew up a terrible stutterer, so I'm about done here, because things could go south at any moment.

But I believe in helping people understand that they are a big part in helping themselves, no matter what cancer, what stage, what age.

The C-word is dreaded and for good reason. But I have chosen to focus on the opening in the letter C. Each and every day, I welcome the blessings and opportunities that flow into the opening, that they may be a part of my plan to impact for the greater good.

My goal is to see myself as whole, and to pass something worthwhile to others. I firmly believe blessings can come from any adversity that we face.

As a certified spiritual director, I believe we are all here to shepherd one another on our spiritual journeys.

Let me close with a quote from Pierre Teilhard de Chardin: "We are not human beings having a spiritual experience. We are spiritual beings having a human experience." Welcome to your experience!

CHAPTER 25

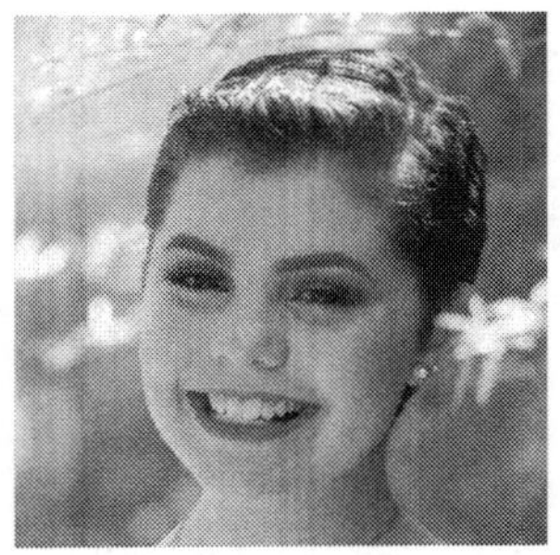

ELIZABETH CAMERON

Ewing's Cancer Survivor

This "one hip wonder" is a 15-year-old cancer survivor making a difference in her community and around the world. Elizabeth is an advocate for childhood cancer, speaking and volunteering with many organiza-tions. She creates makeup bags for girls in the hospital who are going through treatment, as well as providing them with Positivity Pouches. Learn more about her at www.LittleGoldWarrior.com.

CHAPTER 25: ELIZABETH CAMERON

Hi, my name is Elizabeth. If you can't tell I'm a little bit on the short side, 4' 7" to be exact, and that's just on my good leg. My dad is 6' 2" and my mom is five feet. She hoped my dad's genes would help her kids be taller. I'm short and my brother was born with dwarfism. It kinda back fired on her.

Around Easter of 2015, I woke up with a slight pain in my leg. At first, I thought to myself, it's a growing pain! I'm finally growing! The pain got worse and I just figured that it was a dance pain. I've been a dancer since I was two, so injuries were bound to happen.

The pain went away but then it returned. And this time, it was so intense that I could no longer walk or do anything. It became so bad that my parents took me to the doctor to get an x-ray. The x-ray showed nothing, so the doctor referred me to physical therapy. After a few sessions, the pain became worse still. The next diagnosis was a problem with my hip flexor.

The physical therapist said he had never seen a hip flexor so tight in someone so young and he recommended I get an MRI. Bad news: the MRI came back showing an egg-sized mass in my hip. They said it could be lymphoma, sarcoma or leukemia.

We then met with the surgeon who assured us it was more than likely a benign tumor and off I went for a biopsy.

He said he would call my parents in a week once he received the results.

During that time, I was in a tremendous amount of pain but we remained positive and convinced ourselves it was benign. So I named the tumor "Bean" for benign.

A week later, my dad received a phone call, not from the surgeon, but from Phoenix Children's Cancer and Blood Center. They told him my tumor was malignant. There goes the name "Bean!"

We met with an oncologist and she told me that I had a rare bone cancer called Ewing's Sarcoma.

She told me I would have nine months of chemotherapy, surgery and possibly radiation. I told the oncologist that I didn't have time to deal with this, and that I would give her three months.

She disagreed, but I didn't let that get me down. I was admitted that day, July 6th, 2015, and that was the start of my roller coaster.

After the first six rounds of chemo, I had a 12-hour surgery, which resulted in the removal of my entire left hip with no replacement. Joint replacements can sometimes cause infections – which I did not need! In addition, I'm hopefully still growing and a hip today may not fit me tomorrow!

I was told I would not be able to dance or do a lot of other things again. I took this as a challenge.

I've always been the type of person who, when you tell me one thing, I most likely will wanna do the opposite. I might have been a little bit of challenging child at times.

I'm sure most people hadn't seen a one hip dancer. I mean, a one hip anything sounds a little weird. I was going to prove them wrong and I did. I may not dance like I used to, but I dance!

I now call myself the "One Hip Wonder." My left leg is three and a half inches shorter than my right, so I have to wear a shoe lift. Its okay because I've accepted it and it's now my friend.

It was a hard 12 months. I spent over 150 nights in the hospital, multiple hours of physical therapy, countless days of being wheeled around the hospital campus from doctor appointment to doctor appointment. There were hours of throwing up, sleepless nights, anxiety, shots, nasty medicine, pain and ER visits.

If you can imagine being sick all the time, then you can understand it wasn't very fun. But I still woke up every morning and told myself, it's okay. There's someone somewhere who has it so much worse than you do. Be thankful that you woke up this morning and are still breathing.

I'm a strong believer that everything happens for a reason. I knew that I had to go through that so that now I can live out my 2nd Act. And I would go through it all over again because from this, I've gained so much perspective and found so many opportunities to make a difference and learn.

I learned that childhood cancer is a very big problem that no one knows about unless you are in this world. I learned that 47 kids are diagnosed every single day, and seven more become angels every day. Not because of their unwillingness to fight this horrible disease, but because there are no more options for them.

Less than 4 percent of federal funding goes to childhood cancer and that's not okay! We are given a harsh chemo regimen that destroys our immune systems and has many long term side effects.

We lose our hair, our eyebrows and our eyelashes. We are either in the hospital or at home sick. No one sees us. There is not enough awareness for childhood cancer.

Since finding out these facts, I have made it my mission to do whatever I can to make a difference and I've only just begun. Makeup was my therapy during treatment. I would tell people, okay no one bother me. I'm worrying about my face right now and that's all.

It was a distraction from how I was feeling and whatever else was going on in my life. It also made me feel better. I mean, I may not have felt good but I looked good! I wanted to give that feeling to others, so I decided to give girls in the hospital all the tools they would need and it would be great.

I have started to create personalized makeup bags for teen girls in local hospitals. My goal is to expand this to hospitals nationwide. I have already started connecting with other organizations to help make this possible.

I have also spoken at several events, sharing my story and spreading awareness about childhood cancer issues.

Another project in my 2nd Act is creating "Personalized Positivity Pouches" with my aunt. These are special IV pole covers that have pouches on the outside to store positive messages. That way, positivity is covering all of your medicines and chemo bags.

I feel this this is important because we need to think that everything going into our bodies is healing. I had a chemo called the "red devil" because it's red and does the most damage to your heart. It comes in a black bag that says, "Caution, hazardous material."

This can scary to little kids, so having a Personalized Positivity Pouch helps them not think about it. I believe that thinking positive thoughts is very powerful.

On my Facebook fan page, I'm the Little Gold Warrior. Obviously, I'm little. Gold is the color of childhood cancer. And I am a warrior.

Look out world, this Little Gold Warrior's 2nd Act has just begun and I plan to do big things!

CHAPTER 26

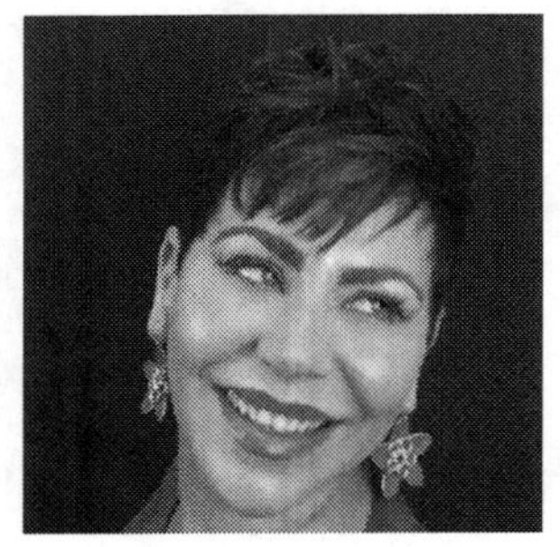

ELANA K. WIGHT

Ovarian Cancer Survivor

Elana is a sixth generation Arizona native and single mother of two high school students. In 2013, she was diagnosed with Stage IV Metastatic Ovarian Cancer. She founded the Red Thursday Foundation, and is also a speaker and business consultant for the professional beauty industry, reaching out to cancer pa-tients and beauty professionals throughout the world.

Learn more at www.RedThursday.org.

Elana Kathryn Wight, and I am a warrior!

On December 12, 2013, after four months of countless doctors visits, my worst fears came true. I had cancer. Not just any cancer but Stage IV Ovarian Cancer. I begin to scream inside.

How can this be? I'm 35. I'm young and vibrant. I'm healthy. I look good! I'm the fun one! This is not me. This isn't happening to me. Cancer happens to "those people." Not me.

What happens to my kids? I'm a single mom. They need me. I've got stuff to do. I have people who depend on me.

Frozen. All I feel is frozen.

Have you ever watched someone with end staged cancer? That's not me. That's not how this goes. That's not my life.

With God's help, I decided to write my own story that day. It would be my personal warrior journey, my mantra about life and not about cancer.

I pulled on my red cowboy boots. I put on my red lipstick, and I went to work: ready to live! I made a conscious choice to share all the details of this journey on social media. I shared my gory, scary, sad and triumphant moments with the world.

I was writing almost every day about my new zeal to live. I decided that each day I had the opportunity to be a better person than the day before, and if it mattered to just one person, then it was worth it.

Chemo after surgery, after surgery after chemo. And brain tumors after brain strokes, and then radiation after surgery after chemo and then more radiation. Drug trials after more chemo, and three times it came back.

Are you listening? It's more than I can explain and more than anyone should endure. But my red boots are still on. I'm smiling with my red lipstick on my lips and I'm still writing my story.

Today I am cancer free.

My red boots and red lipstick helped mold my 2nd Act. When I went through treatment the first time, I had chemo every week on Thursday. I wore my red cowboy boots and put on my red lipstick.

My friends came to chemo with me. We started sharing our weekly pictures of our chemo parties on Facebook and people began to notice. We were having fun! Imagine that? Who has fun at chemo? I do!

And it happened. More people joined me and started wearing red each Thursday.

They posted their own photos to show support to me

and to other cancer patients in their lives. We were seeing posts from all over the world. People noticed life. Thursday became the day to celebrate life, friendship and love.

Red was the color, not because I chose it, but because of all the different emotions it evokes: love, anger, beauty, and courage. Even Ulta Beauty would sell out of "F-Bomb" red lipstick! People loved it, this movement of ours.

My tiny spark became the fire that is now Red Thursday. It went from a social media movement to a small tribe of friends, and last year, only two and half years into this warrior's journey, I was able to create the Red Thursday Foundation.

It is my life's work, my 2nd Act and the divine purpose that God created me to do. I'm reaching as many cancer patients as possible and sharing my warrior journey.

Last year the Red Thursday Foundation hit several milestones. For my 38th birthday, April 28th we delivered red roses to over 300 cancer patients receiving treatment that day.

It was my birthday wish to celebrate life with as many patients as possible. Then, on September 29th, we had our first fundraising gala event.

Last year, I counseled over 250 cancer patients who

reached out to me personally. I have held more hands during chemo than I can count. I cry with them and then I make then laugh by being me, the crazy red head.

We are all in this together. We deliver food and supplies to anyone who asks. I'll talk to anyone who needs us. Our mission is to encourage, inspire and share hope for cancer patients and their caregivers. We believe Red Thursday can be celebrated by everyone, because today, everyone knows someone with cancer.

2017 is going to be an epic year for the Red Thursday Foundation. My goal for Red Thursday is to be used however we can for the advocacy of cancer patients in Arizona.

Last month on Valentine's Day, we delivered marula oil lip balms, specially packaged with our contact info on them so those patients can reach out to us for help in their journey. Our goal is to deliver another 20,000 throughout 2017. Twenty thousand lips is 20,000 happy hearts with hope. And hope saves lives.

I hope to personally make contact with at least half of those patients. I also look for other service opportunities where Red Thursday can partner with organizations to aid them for the support of patients.

There is one more gift cancer brought me. Beyond my 2nd Act, and the crazy red head is Elana. For the first time in my life, I can say I really like her. I am proud to be her. I want to be her friend. She is exactly what the Lord created her to be, and she will never stop living!

CHAPTER 27

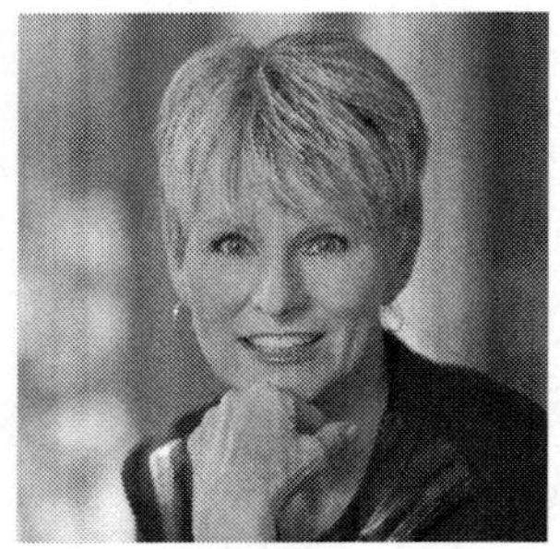

JUDY PEARSON

Triple Negative Breast Cancer Survivor

Judy is a writer, speaker, and the founder of A2ndAct.org. She exists happily – loving each day more than the last – at the foot of the Phoenix Mountain Preserve with her husband, David, and their rescued chocolate lab, Izzy Belle.

CHAPTER 27: JUDY PEARSON

My life felt good. My sons had grown into fine men, although my mommy nerves were on edge as my eldest was about to deploy to Afghanistan.

I had just married the man of my dreams. My emotional plate was full. And then I heard the words that change a life: you have cancer. Triple Negative Breast Cancer. Very aggressive, needing very aggressive treatment.

This couldn't be coming at a worse time, I told my doctor. Her stare said it all. Does cancer ever come at a good time?

Like all the stories you hear, my cancer, too, was a terrifying tornado with me in the middle. I was a control freak losing control with so many questions swirling in my mind.

Would my new husband leave me? Would my son be killed in Afghanistan? Would I die right here at home? I endured surgery - yes they're fake, the real ones tried to kill me and 18 rounds of chemo.

At the end of it all, I fully expected the old Judy would pop out of the chemo cake. But she was no where to be found.

Replacing her was a sweat-drenched, pain-laden, fatigued insomniac, with maniacal tendencies. I asked my doctor why I hadn't been prepared for life after treatment. Her response was to offer me more drugs to counteract those already coursing through my system.

And an even bigger question was born: How could it be that after all a survivor goes through, even after she defeats the beast, she still finds herself dragging its carcass behind her? What's the point of fighting to live if you can't make good use of the life you've been given?

In the five years since my diagnosis, I've met brilliant luminaries in the cancer world. They're working diligently to better treat and cure this dreadful disease. But even if cancer was cured tomorrow, we would still be survivors, still trying to make sense of our journey and define its purpose in our lives.

I've also met thousands of women survivors and I'm overwhelmed by the courageous things many are doing as a payback to society, using their gifts of time and experience. In helping others, they're healing themselves.

There are more than 15 million cancer survivors in this country, eight million of which are women, more than 400,000 of whom live right here in the Valley. We don't need a law or a constitutional amendment to give us our pre-cancer lives back. Most of us like our post cancer lives better anyway!

We simply need to hear one another's stories. They

give us the strength to create 2nd Acts. One by one, we will inspire each other. I created A2ndAct.org to give these stories a vehicle from which to grow. But that little branch has developed into an amazing tree.

We launched a blog, featuring stories of women around the country. We published a book, an ever-growing collection of the stories of the women who have graced our stages. It is always available at every performance of "A 2nd Act: Survivorship Takes the Stage," with that cast's stories included. We host survivor events for the sheer pleasure of networking and hanging out with sister survivors.

We make micro grants to women survivors ready to launch their 2nd Acts, but who are in need of a little seed money. These grants are made in the cities where our performances are held, so the money raised in a city, stays in a city.

And beginning in 2017, we will offer A 2nd Act Workshops, free of charge, to hospitals, treatment facilities, and more. These workshops will guide other survivors to discover their 2nd Acts, in very much the same way each of us discovered ours.

The exponential growth from all of this will have a massive effect, not only among cancer survivors, but for anyone who has faced a life challenge. These 2nd Act stories provide the cast members with a platform to help grow their 2nd Acts. They are our new drugs and will help us live our best lives in the time we have left. I mean truthfully, we're all terminal. Even all of you!

Everything we do has a single purpose: to help survivors change their life question from "Why me?" to "What next?" I am humbled by the love and support – financially and emotionally – our organization has been shown. I am honored and will be eternally grateful. Because, you see, THIS is my 2nd Act.

Made in the USA
San Bernardino, CA
16 February 2017